Vestibular Rehabilitation Therapy for the Patient with Dizziness and Balance Disorders

EXERCISE PROTOCOLS

By

Marian Girardi, Ph.D.

with

Randolph A. McKenzie, M.D.

and

Meiho Nakayama, M.D., Ph.D.

Published by Vestibular Technologies Publications.
www.vestibtech.com

Book design by Pine Orchard Inc.
www.pineorchard.com

Printed in Canada.

ISBN-10: 0-9767593-8-1
ISBN-13: 978-09767593-8-6

Library of Congress Control Number: 2005925161

This book is dedicated to
HORST R. KONRAD, M.D.
teacher, mentor, colleague, and friend.

IN MEMORY

Author MARIAN GIRARDI suddenly passed away in January of 2005, shortly after approving the cover design of her book.

Although she will no longer be able to experience the satisfaction of teaching clinicians or of helping balance-disordered and falls-risk patients, her legacy of compassionate caring, particularly for the elderly, will be forever preserved through the publication and distribution of this book.

Even though she will be sorely missed by her friends and colleagues, her writing ensures that Dr. Marian Girardi will always live on because her words will help improve the quality of life for people all over the world for many, many years to come.

TABLE OF CONTENTS

CHAPTER 1
EXERCISE PROTOCOLS

INTRODUCTION AND SCOPE

According to studies from the National Institutes of Health (NIH 1993), approximately 6 million Americans annually seek medical help because of balance problems and/or vertigo symptoms, and an estimated 90 million Americans (>40% of the current population) will complain to their physicians of dizziness at least once in their lifetimes. Balance disorders and dizziness are among the three most common reasons for elderly individuals to visit a physician, and these disorders are highly significant risk factors for falls in the aging population. It has been estimated that falls are the leading cause of death from injuries in those over 65 years of age as well as the leading cause for death and disability for individuals over the age of 75 (Shepard and Telian 1996). Individuals over age 65 who deny major health problems or acute balance disorders report fall rates exceeding 40% annually; half the people in this age group who fall will fall at least once more within 12 months.

While the etiologies and diagnoses for dizziness and balance disorders include peripheral and central vestibular deficits, presbystasis, strokes and vascular insufficiencies, viral infections, chemical and drug exposures, systemic disorders, head trauma, and anxiety disorders, it is estimated that approximately 85% of these cases are the result of disorders involving the vestibular system (NIH 1993). The cost to society of these vestibular disorders and their accompanying deficits in terms of medical expenses, lost productivity, and patient discomfort and suffering is undetermined, but highly significant. The American Academy of Orthopedic Surgeons estimates direct costs for a hip replacement to be >$40,000. The patient population with vestibular disorders and balance dysfunction represents a highly consequential and often under-served group which frequently can greatly benefit from treatment with Vestibular Rehabilitation Therapy (VRT).

IDENTIFYING THE BALANCE DISORDERED PATIENT

The traditional method of identifying the balance disordered patient has been to wait for such patients to present to their physician with complaints or symptoms of dizziness, vertigo, oscillopsia, loss of balance or disequilibrium. Conscientious physicians would then order or conduct a work-up of the patient which would often result in a referral for VRT. Fortunately, as more and more physicians have become aware of the benefits of VRT in recent years, the incidence of referrals for such treatment has increased greatly. Still, informed therapists and other clinicians have long recognized that the great majority of balance disorder patients are never identified until a fall occurs, when it is often too late for effective intervention.

In an effort to address that issue, in April 2001, the Board of Directors of the American Geriatrics Society approved a new clinical practice guideline, *Guideline for the Prevention of Falls in Older Persons* (AGS 2001), formulated by a special joint committee of the American Geriatrics Society, British Geriatrics Society, and the American Academy of Orthopaedic Surgeons. The Guideline states: "Frequently, older people are not aware of their risks of falling, and neither recognize risk factors nor report these issues to their physicians. Consequently, opportunities for prevention of falling are often overlooked with risks becoming evident only after injury and disability have already occurred" (AGS 2001). The Guideline recommends that all physicians routinely assess all older patients for risk of falling and institute gait and balance therapy.

Unfortunately, most physicians, particularly the primary care physicians who see the largest number of patients, do not have the expertise or the time to properly assess their patients for falls risk by using subjective assessment techniques. Further complicating the process is the fact that most physicians are uncomfortable working with subjective assessments because subjective assessments can only provide them with subjective results. Most physicians prefer to work with objective, quantified results that incorporate normative data based on recognized criteria. Because of such factors, the overwhelming majority of balance disorder/falls risk patients remain unidentified.

A new patent-pending technology, Comprehensive Assessment of Postural Systems (CAPS™), is now being introduced to physicians, therapists, and other clinicians. Designed specifically to quickly identify the at-risk patient, CAPS™ uses a sensitive diagnostic force plate platform and special software (ScreenTRAK™) to assess balance function in 60 seconds by incorporating a computer-based data acquisition system to monitor and record patient movements. Data is acquired while the patient's eyes are closed and his or her proprioceptive input is significantly reduced. Reduction of proprioceptive input is achieved through the use of a specially constructed foam that changes the compliance of the surface on which the patient is standing. The combination of closed eyes and perturbed surface effectively deprives the patient of two of the three sensory inputs, causing the patient to rely almost solely on his or her vestibular system to maintain balance.

The position of the subject's center of gravity over a period of time is used to compute amplitude, speed, and power spectrum of the minute swaying motions of the patient's body; and to calculate maximum sway, stability, predominant direction of sway, directionality of sway, fatigue ratio, and adaptation ratio. Then the information from that patient is compared to a database of age-matched normative data obtained from a large pool of subjects (Amin et al. 2000). The CAPS™ ScreenTRAK™ software then generates a report that graphs the results and classifies the patient's balance/falls risk as "Normal," "Mildly Impaired," "Moderately Impaired," "Severely Impaired," or "Profoundly Impaired."

The report also recommends a focused history, physical evaluation, visual acuity test, and hearing test for patients whose balance falls into the Moderately, Severely, or Profoundly Impaired categories, and advises the physician that the chance of a false positive in such cases is extremely remote. After patients have been diagnosed, the CAPS™ ScreenTRAK™ software may be used to measure therapy progress or to aid in documenting therapy outcomes.

ANATOMY & PHYSIOLOGY
OF THE VESTIBULAR SYSTEM

Adaptive and compensatory mechanisms that are found in the brain and in the inner ear are the basis for VRT. The restoration of normal vestibular mechanisms through physical medicine interventions is utilized as well. VRT takes advantage of these "plastic" characteristics of the CNS to reestablish homeostasis of the entire vestibular system, which results in the fine-tuning of ocular motor skills, amplification of vestibulo-ocular reflex (VOR) control, and improvements in balance, postural control, and movement strategies (Konrad et al. 1992).

When designing an appropriate VRT program for a patient, several other factors must be taken into consideration. The extent and efficacy of the therapy may be limited by the degree and location of damage to the vestibular system and the remaining functional elements. Other important aspects include the capacities of other sensory systems, since vision, proprioception, and to a lesser degree hearing, also play major roles in balance function. Also influencing recovery are the integrity of central systems and physical integrity and motor skills abilities, since skeletal and muscle strength and joint mobility may limit range of motion and activity levels. Additional factors that affect the outcomes of a VRT program include general physical health, decision-making and cognitive abilities, age, memory, and the presence of psychological and anxiety disorders (Herdman 1994).

There are five individual organelles that make up the vestibular apparatus of each inner ear: three semi-circular canals (superior, posterior, and horizontal) and two otolith organs (utricle and saccule). The semi-circular canals in the two ears are paired between ears and function to sense rotary or angular motion, while the otolith organs detect linear accelerations, the primary of these forces being gravity.

Complex neuronal circuits in multiple areas of the brain function to process incoming data from the vestibular, visual, and proprioceptive inputs. The most important of these are the four vestibular nuclei (superior, medial, lateral, and descending), located in the pons and extending into the medulla. Although rapid eye movements are generated in the frontal and parietal cortex regions of the brain, they also require information from visual fields and the occipital cortex. Areas of the cerebellum, the superior colliculus, and the midbrain are also involved in balance maintenance, mainly through the cervical ocular reflex and the vestibulo-spinal reflex.

ASSESSMENT OF THE PATIENT

An accurate diagnosis of the patient, including the location and degree of damage to the peripheral and central vestibular structures and the ancillary balance senses, is of paramount importance when designing a successful VRT program. **The most significant areas to address with therapy are the systems that show altered function during vestibular testing.** Modern diagnostic techniques combine tests of the vestibular system and balance function, a thorough history, and a clinical evaluation. The purpose of balance function testing is generally considered three-fold:

1) to determine the site of lesion and degree of damage to sensory systems and neural pathways;

2) to gather information regarding functional abilities and the use of integrated sensory information; and

3) to evaluate the level of physiological and neuro-otological compensation that may already have occurred (Shepherd 1994).

Electronystagmography (ENG) testing can elicit information on the function of the central and peripheral vestibular systems, using either EOG electrodes or infrared video (Girardi 1997).

Central vestibular function is tested by examining and recording spontaneous and/or gaze-evoked nystagmus and by studying the ocular motor reflexes (saccade, pursuit, and optokinetic). Other tests in the overall ENG battery include investigating positional/positioning provoked nystagmus and vestibular end-organ sensitivity (with caloric and rotational testing). Examination and quantification of the VOR response involve rotational testing. Head autorotation testing at physiological frequencies from 0.5 Hz up to about 6.0 Hz is the preferred modality because it can aid in the diagnosis of central vs. peripheral findings by documenting fixation suppression of movement provoked nystagmus. Caloric testing, the only test modality that isolates information from each inner ear on an individual basis, involves rotation of the endolymphatic fluid in the semicircular canals at a much lower frequency (about 0.003 Hz).

Computer dynamic platform posturography (CDP) is utilized to measure the interrelationship of vision, proprioception, and vestibular systems by assessing sway and/or fall patterns in specific sensory conditions. Also known as Sensory Organization Testing (SOT), the testing protocols involve coupling complete vision and lack of vision with firm and pertubated footings (Jacobson et al. 1993).

Limits of Stability (LOS) testing is used to evaluate the actual stable area of support of the patient, i.e., the area in which the patient's center of gravity must fall in order for the patient to avoid losing balance and falling. A battery of audiological testing may elicit information regarding hearing function, since hearing ability and balance function show a high degree of correlation due to the close proximity of the auditory and vestibular structures. In fact, specific audiological findings may be associated with particular vestibular disorders, i.e., a fluctuating low frequency sensory neural hearing loss and tinnitus often accompany Meniere's disease. Other physiological laboratory tests are frequently required to determine the differential diagnosis of the balance disorder, as many systemic diseases (diabetes, ischemic disorders, migraine, auto-immune diseases, central demyelinating disorders, and cardiovascular diseases) may also present with symptoms similar to vestibular problems.

Results from each of the CDP test batteries give the examiner information regarding a patient's stability and potential risk of falling. By visualizing the patient's sway patterns and examining numerical and graphical results for the LOS tests, the clinician can gather valuable information on the patient's use (or lack of use) of lower body (ankle, hip, and stepping) strategies. These data are of considerable value when designing a customized therapy program for the patient.

A thorough patient history is of paramount importance not only when diagnosing a specific vestibular dysfunction but also when designing a VRT program for a dizzy or balance-disordered patient. In addition to a complete medical history, at minimum the patient should be questioned regarding the onset of current symptoms, an account of previous problems, and the type of symptoms experienced (vertigo, imbalance, disequilibrium, pre-syncopal sensations, gait ataxia, etc.). The frequency and duration of symptoms, any specific activities, and/or positions which provoke symptoms and the presence of oscillopsia or other vision disturbances should be obtained. It is also important to determine the patient's perception of his or her problems with the contributory effects to limiting lifestyle activities. The existence of other otologic symptoms, such as hearing loss, tinnitus, and aural fullness and pressure can also be of use in localization of the lesion.

As the assessment is continued, a complete list of prescription and over-the-counter medications should be obtained since many pharmaceuticals can cause dizziness symptoms, while others may interfere with test results and/or reduce the effectiveness of VRT (Krenning et al. 1996). A recent study at SIU School of Medicine showed that the elderly individual at risk of falling was taking an average of 6.5 prescription medications and 3.5 OTC drugs (Krishna et al. 2004). Determination of the patient's physical status should be made, including measures of range of motion, strength, pain complaints, sensation, proprioception, and coordination.

Vision should also be evaluated and correctable vision abnormalities referred for treatment. Clinicians with access to the CAPS™ Base + Vision system can use the included ScreenTRAK™ visual acuity module software to test the patient's corrected vision by doing a "Tumbling E" Snellen's test of each eye at intermediate distance (6'). The software then scores the patient's visual acuity using conventional terminology, i.e., 20/20; 20/50; 20/200; etc. Dynamic visual acuity testing, which is particularly useful in indicating a bilateral peripheral problem, may be performed if individuals complain of oscillopsia. (See Appendix for Snellen Chart.) If ocular motor studies were not previously performed as part of an ENG test, at a minimum the clinician should do observational testing, including spontaneous and gaze-evoked nystagmus tests, saccade and pursuit studies, and visual-vestibular interactions.

When results from CDP are not available, more traditional balance and postural tests may be performed, including active and passive sitting and standing sway testing, static and dynamic balance testing (Romberg, sharpened Romberg, standing on one leg with eyes open [SOLEO] and with eyes closed [SOLEC] and Fukuda stepping tests).

A substitute for posturography is the modified Clinical Test of Sensory Interaction in Balance (CTSIB). Dynamic movement testing (marching in place and walking with head in motion, quick stops, and turns, etc.) is of great importance in determining gait abnormalities. The Berg Balance Test and Tinetti Balance and Gait tests are highly useful, as is the Functional Reach Test (Herdman 1994). For quick assessment of less mobile patients, Chair Rising, Get Up and Go, and Timed Up and Go tests may be used. All these tests, as well as a thorough assessment form, may be found in the Appendix.

It is not necessary to perform every possible test listed on the form for each patient. Instead, the clinician should limit the test battery to the tasks that will provide the best information regarding the patient's specific complaints (balance, gait, movement, positions, etc.). Physical therapy and occupational therapy intake forms are also available in the Appendix for use as part of the assessment because the vast majority of patients who require VRT therapy also require additional PT and OT services.

Additionally, an analysis of positioning and positionally provoked vertigo should be performed as part of the VRT assessment (Herdman 1994). A survey form involving quality-of-life questions and activities-of-daily-living inquiries can also be very helpful and may be utilized as an objective measurement of the efficacy of a VRT program by having the patient complete the questionnaire(s) prior to and immediately following the completion of the therapy program. The Dizziness Handicap Inventory (DHI) (Jacobsen and Newman 1990) is found in the Appendix.

An assessment form which addresses home safety issues is an important part of the patient intake, and a sample form is in the Appendix. Often changes in environmental conditions that reduce falls-risk factors can be suggested to the patient and/or caregiver. Assessment of the patient's mental state is also of importance in determining if the patient is a candidate for home-based therapy or if in-house rehabilitation will be required. A mini-mental exam is provided in the Appendix for such use.

There are a number of complaints described by patients who are referred for VRT that should raise concerns about diagnoses that are not appropriately addressed with VRT. Patients with many neurological (undiagnosed CNS disease), cardiovascular (brainstem TIA or CVA, basilar migraine), and similar systemic disorders (acoustic neuroma) should be referred to an appropriate physician. Some of the symptoms not related to vestibular disorders include tingling, numbness, and weakness sensations in the extremities; slurred speech; poor coordination and tremors; loss of consciousness; cranial nerve dysfunction; and visual field loss and hearing loss (Herdman 2000).

PATIENT POPULATION FOR VRT

VRT should be considered as a primary treatment modality for patients with any stable vestibular dysfunction for which the symptoms have not been completely resolved by the natural compensatory processes (Shepard and Telian 1995). Individuals with an unstable lesion, usually indicative of a progressive degenerative process, are frequently not good VRT candidates. Patients with fluctuating disorders who exhibit spontaneous vertigo episodes, such as those with endolymphatic hydrops, Meniere's disease, superior canal dehiscence syndrome, or perilymphatic fistula should not be treated with VRT as their primary treatment modality. Patients with vertigo or dizziness symptoms from a demyelinating disease, epilepsy, and migraine are examples of individuals with an unstable central vestibular disorder who are not good VRT candidates. However, VRT modalities, while not treating these specific disorders, may be useful in stabilizing balance for these individuals between episodes. Individuals with vertebrobasilar vascular insufficiencies may present with symptoms of vertigo and nystagmus as well as diplopia, ataxia, dysarthria, and dysphagia. While VRT is not a solution to the vascular blockage, it may assist in improving balance for these individuals.

While patients with CNS lesions or a mixed peripheral etiology may have a more limited prognosis than the patient suffering from a peripheral vestibular problem, these individuals should not be excluded from a VRT program (Shepard and Telian 1995). Persons with multi-factorial balance deficits, such as geriatric patients with a presbystasis diagnosis, may benefit greatly from VRT, particularly when their therapy involves conditioning, postural control, gait and balance exercises.

Additionally, counseling regarding safety issues involving activities of daily living, particularly areas involving falls risks and other issues regarding home-based living, is highly helpful to this patient population (Smith-Wheelock et al. 1992), as is counseling to prevent or combat "fear of falling" syndrome. And by improving overall balance for this population of elderly individuals, the risk of falling may be reduced (Krishna et al. 2004).

TREATMENT WITH VRT

After establishing a diagnosis and completing the VRT assessment of the patient, a customized exercise program can be designed. In order to achieve maximum efficacy in improving balance, diminishing vertigo, and reestablishing equilibrium, current VRT modalities are tailored for the specific individual on the basis of precise diagnostic findings (Shepard and Telian 1995). A number of studies have shown that customized VRT programs are significantly more efficacious in resolving symptoms than generic exercises (Smith-Wheelock et al. 1991A).

VRT is no longer considered a final, desperate treatment when pharmacological and/or surgical options fail; but, in fact, VRT is frequently the best and should be considered the first, therapeutic modality for many disorders. This is due to the foundation of VRT that involves utilizing the normal, established adaptive mechanisms already at work in the patient's CNS. Many current program paradigms utilize a therapist-directed, patient-motivated, home-based exercise protocol where individuals visit the therapist on a limited basis and perform their specifically designed exercises at home, without therapist supervision, several times each day, reporting to the therapist at regular visits. Depending upon the individual's specifics, such return visits to the therapist may be on a weekly, bi-weekly, or even more infrequent basis.

Approximately 10-15 minutes is needed to perform each exercise regimen, with a minimum of one to two minutes needed for each individual exercise, and never more than five individual exercises in each regimen. The VRT exercises are graduated, beginning at the minimal skill levels which the patient is capable of performing and then gradually increasing in complexity as compensation and habituation increase and cause provoked and spontaneous symptoms to decrease. If the patient is considered to be at a high risk for falling, or in some other way not capable of performing a home-based self-directed program, out-patient therapy with frequent visits to the therapist at the clinic is recommended. And on some occasions, therapy administered by home-health personnel may be necessary.

BENIGN PAROXYSMAL POSITIONAL VERTIGO

Of the many diagnoses for which VRT serves as an appropriate treatment modality, patients with benign paroxysmal positional vertigo (BPPV) are the most amenable to therapy. This is especially true for individuals with stable BPPV disorders who experience persistent symptoms and lack any central vestibular deficits. Efficacy approaches 100% in several studies for these patients (Herdman et al. 1993). Several single treatment approaches for BPPV, such as the Liberatory Maneuver (Semont et al. 1988), the Canalith Repositioning Procedure (Epley 1992), and numerous modified versions of these treatments are available in the otolaryngology literature (Girardi and Konrad 1996). There are also several multiple treatment approaches that have been published, but with generally lower efficacies. For all approaches, however, the scientific basis for the therapy involves the movement of debris particles (thought to be displaced otoconia) from the long arm of one of the semi-circular canals (usually the posterior) through the common crus into the utricle.

Patients with this disorder are diagnosed by history and physical findings: when placed in the head-hanging left or right (Dix-Hallpike) position, following a brief delay, a short burst of transitory vertigo occurs which is accompanied by a torsional nystagmus. Symptoms characteristically last less than one minute and fatigue upon multiple repeats of the provoking position. It is relatively common for patients to experience disequilibrium and loss-of-balance symptoms following a successful BPPV maneuver if other central or peripheral vestibular involvement is present. These ancillary symptoms usually respond well to other types of VRT. Chapter 4 contains a more detailed description of this disorder and its various treatments.

UNILATERAL PERIPHERAL VESTIBULAR LOSS

Individuals who have an uncompensated unilateral peripheral vestibular lesion generally have an excellent prognosis for recovery from their vestibular symptoms with VRT intervention. A recent study showed greater than 90% of individuals in this category who did not have additional complications from head injury recovered from their symptoms within a matter of several weeks (Shephard et al. 1993). Some common examples of patients with an uncompensated unilateral vestibular dysfunction are persons with vestibular labyrinthitis or neuritis; post-surgical patients who have undergone vestibular nerve section or small acoustic neuroma removal; individuals who have had an inadvertent surgical trauma, a closed head trauma involving injury to the Templar bone; or patients for whom a chemical (streptomycin/gentamycin) labyrinthectomy was performed. For these patients, VRT should be begun at the earliest opportunity following the injury since later intervention may result in incomplete recovery (Smith-Wheelock et al. 1991B).

The exercises for these individuals should include head movements in all three planes with and without visual fixation. They should be started as soon as possible following the onset of symptoms and continue until symptoms have been extinguished. The head movements should mirror the movements which cause the patient to be symptomatic, so patients should be warned that there is a crescendo/decrescendo effect where their symptoms may worsen before they improve and that they may experience an exacerbation of symptoms when performing the exercises, particularly early in the therapy regime.

BILATERAL PERIPHERAL VESTIBULAR LOSS

Uncompensated bilateral vestibulopathy patients are also good candidates for treatment with VRT. A recent study showed 50% of bilateral vestibular paresis patients reporting improvement in symptoms after performing customized VRT exercises (Krebs et al. 1993). The most commonly seen etiology for these individuals is chemical ototoxicity, usually as a result of aminoglycoside antibiotics (particularly streptomycin and gentamycin), industrial solvents (mainly aromatic hydrocarbons), and oncological chemotherapeutic agents (cisplatinin). These patients usually do not complain of vertigo symptoms, since damage to the vestibular end-organs is bilateral and there is no asymmetry in vestibular function. Instead, they usually present with symptoms of a loss of balance, gait ataxia, oscillopsia and a visual dependence which manifests itself in an inability to function in dark conditions.

However, patients who have had a unilateral peripheral vestibular loss in the past may complain of vertigo if the remaining functional ear becomes affected. Substitution exercises are important for these individuals to teach them effective utilization of the other two primary sensory inputs: vision and proprioception. Often these patients become overly dependent on visual input, which can put them at an increased risk of falling in situations where vision is reduced. Substitution exercises encourage more accurate inputs from the proprioceptive sense. These exercises are designed to reduce the usage of visual inputs while gradually increasing somatosensory inputs for postural orientation. Balance exercises should be performed with gradually lowered lighting, increasing textures in the flooring, and equilibrium-requiring activities in visually more complex environments.

For these individuals, balance exercises aid in improving postural control and gaze stabilization exercises with head movements, serve to elicit improvement in dynamic visual acuity and dynamic movement strategy exercises, and ameliorate gait dysfunctions and motor skills deficits.

OTHER DISORDERS

Closed head trauma patients may also present with vestibular symptoms. While they frequently respond well to VRT for their dizziness and balance symptoms, often other central involvement is present and a multidisciplinary head trauma rehabilitative program should be considered in addition to the VRT. Anxiety disordered patients are another category of individuals who may exhibit vestibular-like symptoms. Panic attacks may be due to abnormalities in brainstem neurons that are involved in autonomic regulatory processes; therefore, many individuals who experience panic attacks frequently complain of dizziness (Klein 1993). VRT is quite often an appropriate modality in some patients with milder to moderate psychogenic dizziness; but intervention and ancillary services from psychology/ psychiatry may be required as well (Jacob 1988).

CENTRAL LESIONS

Patients with a stable lesion in the central vestibulo-ocular pathways should also be considered candidates for a VRT program; however, the length of time involved with VRT is usually significantly longer for these patients when compared to those with a peripheral lesion (Shumway-Cook and Horak 1990). Individuals with a central lesion frequently complain of imbalance and disequilibrium rather than vertigo. Persons with such lesions caused by the normal aging process show a poor performance on ocular motor testing. Their results may show an increase in saccade latencies and a decrease in pursuit gains; and a low intensity, sub-clinical threshold, direction-fixed nystagmus may appear throughout the entire ENG test battery. Pure vertical nystagmus seen in any test is always indicative of a central lesion. Exercises involving eye-tracking movements of sinusoidal pursuit; saccade movements in the horizontal, vertical, and lateral planes; and head/eye coordination exercises frequently aid in improvement of these ocular motor reflexes. Individuals with age-related cerebellar atrophy or comparable presbystasis changes that result in increased disequilibrium symptoms respond well to coordination, balance, and motor-skills exercises (Smith-Wheelock et al. 1991A).

Ancillary disorders which may contribute to unsteadiness; lack of coordination and imbalance, such as brainstem small vessel ischemia; other circulatory/vascular disease; or diabetic peripheral neuropathy may also be present in the balance disorder patient. For these individuals, physical therapy modalities (strength training, reaction time maneuvers, stretching, and increased sensory input gait and balance exercises) may be required in addition to VRT, and referral is recommended.

COMBINED ETIOLOGY PATIENTS

Another group of patients referred for VRT is individuals with mixed peripheral and central vestibular findings. This combined etiology group usually demonstrates a poorer overall success rate when compared to the other "single" diagnosis groups (Girardi and Konrad 1998). As described previously, these individuals should be treated with exercises for both the peripheral and the central lesion, depending on the results of their assessment.

BALANCE DISORDER PATIENTS

It is not uncommon for patients to have perfectly normal ENG test results while having poor performance scores on CAPS™ or other posturography tests. This is particularly true in elderly individuals with multi-sensory deficits. In one study involving a population of elderly patients who had fallen at least once, roughly one-half had positive results on one test modality and negative results on the other (Girardi et al. 2001). The reason for the poor balance and falls risk for these individuals is commonly due to loss of lower body motor strategies that are used for equilibrium.

When a mild perturbation of balance occurs, an ankle strategy is correctly used to retain an upright posture. This involves movement at the ankle without movement of the hips and knees. Also, a stronger perturbation elicits a hip strategy response where the individual bends at the hips. With aging, these more primary responses are lost, with the result that even the mildest perturbation involves using a stepping strategy. Due to the increase in reaction time that advanced age may bring about, by the time the patient relocates the stepping leg, a fall has often already occurred.

To improve and promote ankle strategies, exercises such as forward-and-backward and side-to-side sway, stepping up, and walking with abrupt stops and rapid pivot turns are utilized. Improvement of hip strategy exercises include toe/heel stance, tandem standing and walking, and walking a narrow line or on a beam. Stepping strategies can be promoted with exercises that move the center of mass outside the base of support.

GAIT DISORDER PATIENTS

It is much more difficult to maintain balance during gait than at a quiet stance. The majority of falls in the elderly population occur at the initiation of or during locomotion. There are several reasons for this. While in motion during the stance phase of the gait cycle, the center of gravity is moved outside the base of support. Roughly 70% of the body's center of mass is located in the upper body and is moving forward with the body's momentum. During walking, 80% of the time is spent in a single limb stance. Some of the most common changes in gait pattern due to aging are slower walking speed, shorter steps, a more broad-based gait and longer time spent in the double support phase of movement. Ataxic gait is correlated with risk of falling in the elderly population as the gait abnormalities are frequently due to balance disorders and not a change in locomotion.

Gait improvement exercises such as walking with the head in motion, carrying items, performing quick stops and turns, and movement around obstacles are designed to address these deficits. Elderly patients frequently avoid movements that would challenge their balance during gait or they accommodate their gait to their loss of balance. Exercises for gait should involve changing visual information and utilization of alternate strategies to avoid and improve gait deficits (Shumway-Cook and Woollcott 1995).

RISK FACTORS FOR FALLING

Personal risk factors account for approximately 75% of the risk of falls and are related to acquired disabilities, age-related changes, and current diseases. The rate of hip fractures increases after age 50, doubling every five to six years. Lack of weight-bearing exercise leads to decreased bone strength. Women fall more often than men, or at least report falling more often. Reduced levels of estrogen after menopause can result in osteoporosis; thus, women have two to three times as many hip fractures as men. Women have a 20% chance of a hip fracture during their lifetimes. Smoking and/or excessive alcohol intake decrease bone strength. Chronic alcohol abuse increases dizziness symptoms with head and body movements and can be responsible for positionally-provoked, alcohol-induced nystagmus (PAN II) which closely resembles BPPV. Caucasians and Asians with small slender body structures are at risk; so are people who have a family history of fractures later in life. Low calcium dietary intake, reduced calcium absorption, and inadequate vitamin D are factors in osteoporosis. Severely decreased caloric intake can cause weakness and contribute to falling.

Medical risk factors also increase the occurrence of falls in the elderly. These include co-morbidity factors such as cardiac arrhythmias (irregular heartbeat), blood pressure fluctuation, and history of stroke. Diabetes mellitus and its resulting complications (peripheral neuropathy, diabetic retinopathy, kidney disease) can lead to loss of proprioception and vision, as well as episodes of light-headedness and presyncopal sensations. Cancer that affects bones can increase the risk of a fracture as a result of a fall. Depression, Alzheimer's disease, senility, cognitive impairment, anxiety and panic disorders—all have been shown to increase the risk of falling and may be the cause of dizziness and balance loss symptoms.

Arthritis and hip or knee weakness can increase imbalance, leading to additional falls risk. Neurologic conditions, strokes, Parkinson's disease, multiple sclerosis can all involve symptoms in which balance is decreased. Urinary and bladder dysfunction can lead to excessive visits to the bathroom, particularly at night, when decreased lighting increases the risk of falling.

Vision and/or hearing loss reduce the sensory inputs needed for balance. Elderly individuals taking four or more medications or any psychoactive medication have been shown to be at a greater risk of falling as many of these medications either have dizziness or balance loss as a side effect, or they depress the reaction time to perturbation in balance.

REDUCTION OF MEDICAL RISK FACTORS

There are a number of ways in which elderly individuals can reduce their medical risk factors, thereby also reducing their risk of falling. They should get an annual physical, including an eye examination and hearing test, and also including an evaluation of cardiac and blood pressure problems, and a balance screening exam. Maintenance of a diet with adequate caloric intake, dietary calcium, and vitamin D is very important, as is participation in an exercise program for agility, strength, balance, and coordination (particularly lower body). These individuals should be advised to keep an up-to-date list of all medications and provide it to all doctors with whom they consult. They should inquire about the side effects of their medications by discussing their prescriptions with a nurse, doctor, or pharmacist. It is important that they make sure all medications are clearly labeled and stored in a well-lit area according to instructions and that all medications are taken on schedule with a full glass of water, unless otherwise instructed. Elderly patients should be sure to discuss with their physician(s) ALL medications taken, both prescription and over-the-counter.

REDUCTION OF OTHER RISK FACTORS

Many falls-risk factors for the elderly involve environmental factors and activities of daily living, and can be addressed by an occupational therapist. Individuals should be reminded to get up slowly and begin moving slowly. They should be advised to select stable chairs with suitable seat height and to walk close to walls whenever possible. They should be highly encouraged to exercise regularly in a controlled environment, with those exercises including head and eye movements. They should be advised to remove raised doorway thresholds in all rooms and to replace all loose rugs and extension cords in open areas.

Avoidance of difficult-to-reach shelves and avoidance of standing on furniture or other items to reach difficult places should be encouraged. They should be reminded to be sure stairways and entryways are well-lit and have sturdy hand-rails or grab handles. They should be told to be sure they have grab handles and nonskid mats outside of showers and tubs, and next to the toilet. They should be cautioned NOT TO USE TOWEL RACKS IN PLACE OF GRAB BARS—towel racks were not designed to take the weight. Since the bedroom is the site of the highest frequency of falls in the home, it is extremely important for elderly persons to put a light switch by the bedroom door and by the bed, or to keep a night light on so they do not have to walk across a dark room. Also, they need to be sure that their bed is of the correct height so it is not necessary for them to strain to climb into bed and so that their feet can easily touch the floor when getting out.

When bending over to pick up an item from the floor, elderly patients should be taught to stabilize themselves with one hand on a wall or a solid piece of furniture. They need to be advised to remove from regularly used walkways any furniture, throw rugs, or other similar items that could clutter up those areas. They should also be advised to wipe up any liquid spills from floors immediately. If necessary, they should be instructed how to use walking aids such as canes or walkers correctly and to seek professional advice if in doubt. They should be encouraged to wear clothing of suitable length and to wear non-slip shoes with low heels. If they have a pet, they need to be warned that they need to be aware of its location at all times and to be careful when visiting others who have pets. It is also a good idea to talk to them about the importance of having adequate lighting throughout their house and around their yard.

FEAR OF FALLING SYNDROME

One of the most serious consequences of falling in the elderly is a psychological complication: the fear of falling syndrome. While other psychological conditions such as depression, anxiety, and poor coping strategies are also prevalent, the fear of falling and its accompanying psychosocial reactions are usually the most severe and debilitating. The cause of this disorder is difficult to isolate and may simply begin as an unpleasant feeling following a fall. It may be complicated by embarrassment, injury, or functional dependency. The result can be an increased sensitivity to the environment, situations, and conditions which lead to the initial fall as well as a reduction in activities of daily living that could possibly precipitate another fall episode. Often, elderly individuals become so preoccupied with fall avoidance that they allow that trepidation to become a controlling factor in their lives. This leads to limited mobility, reduced fitness, and decreased balance—all of which, in turn, increase falls risks (Tideiksaar 1997).

Experts now recommend that an assessment to delineate the presence and extent of fear of falling should accompany the initial patient evaluation for therapy. While the therapist can simply question the patient and/or family members about such fears, it is not uncommon for the elderly to deny such symptoms or suppress their importance to avoid a decrease in their autonomy. The single question that is most predictive of confident performance is: "Do you need assistance to ambulate out of doors?" The "Activities-Specific Balance Confidence (ABC) Scale" is one instrument developed to quantitatively determine an individual's fear of falling (Powell and Myers 1995). It has been shown that falls are directly related to the ABC score with excellent test/retest reliability. A copy is available in the Appendix.

Once identified, the therapist should attempt to reduce this fear-of-falling cycle. VRT exercises for improved balance and increased strength may improve mobility and increase confidence levels. For some patients, an ancillary device, such as a cane or walker that provides visual and proprioceptive support, can decrease fear of falling, particularly early in the therapy program. As the patient develops increased balance and more confidence, the use of such devices can be gradually reduced. Improving the patient's environment by reducing falls risk can lead to an amelioration of fears. Confidence-building items, such as the installation of grab bars in the bathroom and ensuring adequate illumination in the residential environment, fall into this category.

Patients need to be encouraged to increase their activities of daily living, performing more tasks without the assistance of a caregiver whenever possible since such activities aid in building their confidence. Following a successful VRT regime, elderly fallers should also be motivated to resume any social activities that they enjoyed prior to falling. These activities could include regular attendance at a senior center or similar activities aimed at elderly individuals, shopping, going to church, or simply taking a walk outdoors. Caregivers and other family members should be encouraged to participate in these activities as well.

CONCLUSION

Although a satisfactory initial compensation for vestibular dysfunctions may readily occur, central vestibular system decompensation may also be seen, sometimes with no evident cause. However, this decompensation usually follows periods of immobility, physical or emotional stress, illness, and/or fatigue. Once it has been recognized that this relapse has not occurred due to progressive vestibular disease or an episodic vestibular disorder, it is highly appropriate to restart the VRT program, generally with the same type of exercises that were effective prior to the decompensation episode.

There is a plenitude of data available in the literature regarding the efficacy of VRT in treating the dizzy and balance-disordered patient (Bauer and Girardi 2000; Coward et al. 1998; Girardi and Konrad 1998; Horak et al. 1991; Konrad et al. 1992; Norre 1987; Shumway-Cook and Horak 1989); but all studies have shown that in order to be effective, exercises must include vision, head and eye movements. Additionally, when enrolled in a VRT program, the patient's use of central and peripheral vestibular-suppressive medications should be limited, as most of those pharmacological agents may actually delay compensation and recovery.

It is important to carefully assess all patients to ascertain which specific movements and conditions elicit their symptoms in order to utilize that information when designing their customized VRT program. Persons with a stable vestibular lesion in the central and/or peripheral vestibular system who complain of vertigo, loss of balance and/or disequilibrium; the elderly with balance and gait deficits; and those individuals with a BPPV diagnosis have a maximal prognosis for recovery when treated with VRT, which should be considered the primary therapeutic modality for these individuals.

REFERENCES

American Geriatrics Society (AGS) Panel on Falls Prevention. 2001. Guideline for the prevention of falls in older persons. *J. Am. Geriatr. Soc.* 49 (May):664-72.

Amin, M., M. Girardi, M.E. Neill, and H.R. Konrad. Feb. 15-19, 1998. ENG results pre- and post-carotid endarterectomy surgery. Presented at the ARO Midwinter Meeting, St. Petersburg Beach, FL. Abstract published in the Abstracts from the 1998 ARO Midwinter Meeting.

Amin, M., M. Girardi, H.R. Konrad, and L.F. Hughes. Sept. 24-27, 2000. Normative data for the Balance Trak 500. Presented at the American Academy of Otolaryngology Head and Neck Surgery Foundation Annual Meeting, Washington, DC. Abstract published in Abstracts of the AAO-HNS 2000 Annual Meeting.

Amin, M., H.R. Konrad, and M. Girardi. 2001. ENG rotational testing. In *E-medicine*, online medical textbook.

Amin, M., M. Girardi, M.E. Neill, H.R. Konrad, and L.F. Hughes. Sept. 2001. Electronystagmography testing: A comparison of electro-oculography and infra-red video. *Eye Dynamics, Inc. Newsletter* 5 (2).

Bauer, C.A., and M. Girardi. 2000. Vestibular rehabilitation. In *E-medicine*, online medical textbook.

Coward, J.L., D.M. Wrisley, M. Walker, B. Strasnick, and J.T. Jacobson. 1998. Efficacy of vestibular rehabilitation. *J. Otol. Head Neck Surg.* 118:49-54.

Epley, J. 1992. The canalith repositioning procedure: For treatment of benign paroxysmal positional vertigo. *J. Otol. Head Neck Surg.* 107:399-402.

Girardi, M. 1997. The use of infrared video goggles for nystagmus testing. *Vestibular Update* (Spring/Summer) no. 18:1-3.

Girardi, M., and H.R. Konrad. 1996. Management of benign paroxysmal positional vertigo. *ORL-Head and Neck Nursing* 14:25-30.

Girardi, M., and H.R. Konrad. 1998. Vestibular rehabilitation therapy for the patient with dizziness and balance disorders. *ORL-Head and Neck Nursing* 16:13-22.

Girardi, M., H.R. Konrad, M. Amin, and L.F. Hughes. 2001. Predicting falls risks in an elderly population: Computer dynamic posturography vs. electronystagmography test results. *Laryngoscope* 111:1528-32.

Girardi, M., M. Amin, H.R. Konrad, L.F. Hughes, L. Hock, and K. Jones. 2004. Medical profile of a group of elderly fallers. *Otology and Neurotology*, accepted for publication.

Herdman, S.J., R.J. Tusa, D.S. Zee, L. Proctor, and D.E. Mattox. 1993. Single treatment approaches to benign paroxysmal positional vertigo. *Arch. Otolaryngol. Head Neck Surg.* 119:450-61.

Herdman, S.J., ed. 1994. *Vestibular rehabilitation.* Philadelphia: F.A. Davis.

Horak, F.B., C. Jones-Rycewicz, F.O. Black, et al. 1991. Effect of vestibular rehab on dizziness and imbalance. *J. Otol. Head Neck Surg.* 106:175-80.

Jacob, R.G. 1988. Panic disorder and the vestibular system. *Psychiatr. Clin. of North Am.* 11:361-74.

Jacobson, G.P., and C.W. Newman. 1990. The development of the dizziness handicap inventory. *Arch. Otolaryngol. Head Neck Surg.* 116:424-427.

Jacobson, G.P., C.W. Newman, and J.M. Kartush. 1993. *Handbook of balance function testing.* New York: Mosby Year Book.

Klein, D.F. 1993. False suffocation alarms, spontaneous panics, and related conditions. *Arch. Gen. Psychiatry* 50:306-17.

Konrad, H.R., D. Tomlinson, C.W. Stockwell, M.E. Norre, F.B. Horak, N.T. Shepard, and S.J. Herdman. 1992. Rehabilitation therapy for patients with disequilibrium and balance disorders. *J. Otol. Head Neck Surg.* 107:105-08.

Krebs, D.E., K.M. Gill-Body, P.O. Riley, and S.W. Parker. 1993. Double-blind, placebo-controlled trial of rehabilitation for bilateral vestibular hypofunction: Preliminary report. *J. Otol. Head Neck Surg.* 109:735-41.

Krenning, J., M. Girardi, and H.R. Konrad. 1996. The effect of drugs on electronystagmography test results. *Vestibular Update* (Summer/Fall) no. 17:1-5.

Krishna, P., M. Amin, H.R. Konrad, S.L. Lin, L.F. Hughes, and M. Girardi. 2004. Efficacy of a falls prevention clinic: A pilot study utilizing quality of life assessments. *OtoNeuroto*, accepted for publication, in press.

National Institute on Deafness and Other Communication Disorders, U.S. Department of Health and Human Services, National Institutes of Health. 1993. The national strategic research plan. Publication no. 95-3711:157-96.

Norre, M.E. 1987. Rationale of rehabilitation treatment for vertigo. *Am. J. Otol.* 8:31-5.

Powell, I.E., and A.M. Myers. 1995. The activities-specific balance confidence (ABC) scale. *J. Gerontol.: A Biol. Sci. Med. Sci.* 50A:M28-34.

Semont, A., G. Freyess, and E. Vitte. 1988. Curing the BPPV with a liberatory maneuver. *Adv. Oto-Rhino-Laryngol* 42:290-93.

Shephard, N.T., S.A. Telian, M. Smith-Wheelock, and A. Raj. 1993. Vestibular and balance rehabilitation therapy. *Ann. Otol Rhinol Laryngol* 102:198-204.

Shepherd, N.T., and S.A. Telian. 1994. Evaluation of balance system function. In *Handbook of clinical audiology.* 4th ed., eds. J. Katz, and R.A. Ruth, 424-27. Baltimore: Willliams & Wilkins.

Shepard, N.T., and S.A. Telian. 1995. Programatic vestibular rehabilitation. *J. Otol. Head Neck Surg.* 112:173-182.

Shepard, N.T., and S.A. Telian. 1996. *Practical management of the balance disorder patient.* San Diego: Singular Publishing Group.

Shumway-Cook, A., and F.B. Horak. 1986. Assessing the influence of sensory interaction of balance. *Physical Therapy* 66:1548-50.

Shumway-Cook, A., and F.B. Horak. 1989. Vestibular rehabilitation: An exercise approach to manage symptoms of vestibular dysfunction. *Semin. Hear.* 10:196-208.

Shumway-Cook, A., and F.B. Horak. 1990. Rehabilitation strategies for patients with vestibular deficits. *Neurology Clinics* 8:441-57.

Shumway-Cook, A., and A. Woollcott. 1995. *Motor control theory and practical applications.* Baltimore: Williams and Wilkins.

Smith-Wheelock, M., N.T. Shepard, and S.A. Telian. 1991A. Physical therapy program for vestibular rehabilitation. *Am. J. Otol.* 12:218-25.

Smith-Wheelock, M., N.T. Shepard, and S.A. Telian. 1991B. Long-term effects for treatment of balance dysfunction: Utilizing a home exercise approach. *Semin. Hear.* 12:297-302.

Smith-Wheelock, M., N.T. Shephard, S.A. Telian, and T. Boismier. 1992. Balance retraining therapy in the elderly. Proceedings of the Otolaryngologic Cherry Blossom Conference. In *Clinical otolaryngologic care of the geriatric patient,* 71-80. Philadelphia: BC Decker.

Tideiksaar, Rein. 1997. *Falling in old age: Prevention and management.* 2nd ed. New York: Springer Publishing.

CHAPTER 2

GAZE STABILIZATION AND VOR ENHANCEMENT EXERCISES

GAZE STABILIZATION

Patients should be given this exercise when their ENG gaze-evoked or spontaneous nystagmus tests show ANY abnormalities. Generally, this means gaze-evoked and/or spontaneous nystagmus of any type: horizontal, vertical, torsional, or oblique that is present and recorded or visualized. It can also include any subjective patient complaints of dizziness or lightheadedness while performing the testing. If the caloric test shows a failure of fixation suppression, this exercise should be given. This exercise should also be given if the patient has subjective complaints with any type of eye or head movements, even if not symptomatic during the testing.

Generally, it is best to start patients sitting and moving their heads in just the horizontal and vertical directions, 15 to 20 repeats in each direction. Progress by moving patient to standing (feet apart, feet together, feet pointed), faster head movements, increased number of repeats, diagonal plane movements, and/or lowered lighting. Also, progress patients by having them move the target card to a busy visual background, such as a checkerboard (available in the Appendix section).

GAZE STABILIZATION

1) This exercise is to be performed _____ repeats.

2) This exercise is to be performed in the:
   ❑ horizontal plane
   ❑ vertical plane
   ❑ diagonal plane

3) This exercise is to be performed:
   ❑ eyes open
   ❑ eyes closed

4) This exercise is to be performed:
   ❑ sitting, supported
   ❑ sitting, unsupported
   ❑ standing, supported and ❑ feet shoulder-width apart ❑ feet together
   ❑ standing, unsupported and ❑ feet shoulder-width apart ❑ feet together

5) Hold the target card 12-18 inches in front of your eyes. Be sure you can focus on the letters on the card.

6) Keeping the card still and your eyes focused on the letters on the card, slowly move your head back and forth (horizontally), left and right. DO NOT MOVE YOUR HEAD SO FAST THAT THE LETTERS BECOME BLURRED OR OUT OF FOCUS!

7) Progress by moving your head in the vertical plane and/or the diagonal plane. Progress by placing the target card in the center of a busy visual background, such as a checkerboard. All progressions should be directed by your therapist. Try to keep increasing the speed that your head is moving. Remember to keep the letters in the card in focus—move only your head.

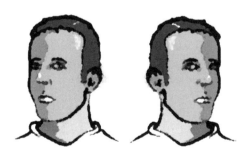

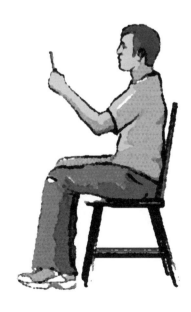

TIMES ONE VIEWING
Target In Phase with Head

Patients should be given this exercise when their auto-rotational VOR testing or caloric tests show ANY abnormalities. This can include significantly increased or decreased gain or phase or increased asymmetry on the auto-rotational VOR testing test, or any subjective patient complaints of dizziness or lightheadedness while performing the testing. This exercise should also be given if the patient has subjective complaints with any type of head and eye movements utilizing the pursuit reflex, even if not symptomatic during the testing.

Generally, it is best to start patients sitting and moving the upper body in just the horizontal and vertical directions, 15 to 20 repeats in each direction. Progress by moving the patient to standing (feet apart, feet together, feet pointed), faster body movements, increased number of repeats, diagonal plane movements, and/or lowered lighting. Also, progress patients by having them move the target card to a busy visual background, such as a checkerboard. (Both card and background are available in the Appendix section.)

TIMES ONE VIEWING
Target In Phase with Head

1) This exercise is to be performed _____ repeats.

2) This exercise is to be performed in the:
   ❑ horizontal plane
   ❑ vertical plane
   ❑ diagonal plane

3) This exercise is to be performed:
   ❑ eyes open
   ❑ eyes closed

4) This exercise is to be performed:
   ❑ sitting, supported
   ❑ sitting, unsupported
   ❑ standing, supported and ❑ feet shoulder-width apart ❑ feet together
   ❑ standing, unsupported and ❑ feet shoulder-width apart ❑ feet together
   ❑ standing on a foam cushion

5) Hold the target card 12-18 inches in front of your eyes. Be sure you can focus on the letters on the card.

6) Slowly move the card left and right (horizontally), keeping your eyes focused on the letters on the target, and moving your entire upper body to go a full 180 degrees. Change hands, if necessary, to keep the card in view at all times. Move the entire upper body (not just your head) to maintain a focus on the letters of the card. DO NOT MOVE THE CARD AND YOUR HEAD SO FAST THAT THE LETTERS BECOME BLURRED OR OUT OF FOCUS!

7) Progress by moving in the vertical plane and/or the diagonal plane. Progress by placing the target card in the center of a busy visual background, such as a checkerboard. All progressions should be directed by your therapist. Try to keep increasing the speed at which the card and your head are moving. Remember to keep the letters in the card in focus and to use your entire upper body, not just your head, to move with the card.

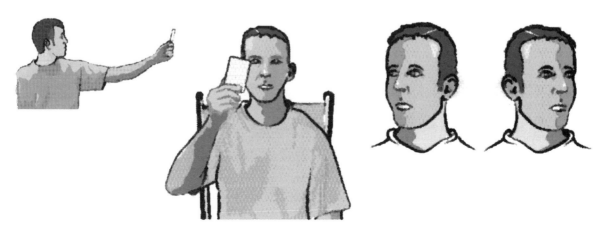

TIMES TWO VIEWING
Target Out of Phase with Head

Patients should be given this exercise when their auto-rotational VOR testing or caloric tests show ANY abnormalities. This can include significantly increased or decreased gain or phase or increased asymmetry on the auto-rotational VOR testing, failure of fixation suppression on the caloric test, or any subjective patient complaints of dizziness or lightheadedness while performing the testing. This exercise should also be given if the patient has subjective complaints with any type of head and eye movements utilizing the pursuit reflex, even if not symptomatic during the testing.

Generally, it is best to start patients sitting and moving their head opposite the target in just the horizontal and vertical directions, 15 to 20 repeats in each direction. Progress by moving the patient to standing (feet apart, feet together, feet pointed), faster body movements, increased number of repeats, diagonal plane movements, and/or lowered lighting. Also, progress patients by having them move the target card to a busy visual background, such as a checkerboard (both available in the Appendix section).

Begin this exercise after the patient can successfully accomplish the Times One Viewing Exercise.

TIMES TWO VIEWING
Target Out of Phase with Head

1) This exercise is to be performed _____ repeats.

2) This exercise is to be performed in the:
   ❑ horizontal plane
   ❑ vertical plane
   ❑ diagonal plane

3) This exercise is to be performed:
   ❑ eyes open
   ❑ eyes closed

4) This exercise is to be performed:
   ❑ sitting, supported
   ❑ sitting, unsupported
   ❑ standing, supported and ❑ feet shoulder-width apart ❑ feet together
   ❑ standing, unsupported and ❑ feet shoulder-width apart ❑ feet together
   ❑ standing on a foam cushion

5) Hold the target card 12-18 inches in front of your eyes. Be sure you can focus on the letters on the card.

6) Slowly move the card left and right (horizontally), keeping your eyes focused on the letters on the target. Move your head in the opposite direction of the card movement. When the card is moved to the left, move your head to the right; when the card is moved to the right, move your head to the left; but make sure your eyes remain focused on the letters on the card at all times. DO NOT MOVE THE CARD OR YOUR HEAD SO FAST THAT THE LETTERS BECOME BLURRED OR OUT OF FOCUS!

7) Progress by moving in the vertical plane (target goes up, head goes down, eyes stay focused on the card, etc.) and/or the diagonal plane. Progress by placing the target card in the center of a busy visual background, such as a checkerboard. All progressions should be directed by your therapist. Try to keep increasing the speed at which you are moving both the card and your head, but remember to keep the letters on the card in focus at all times.

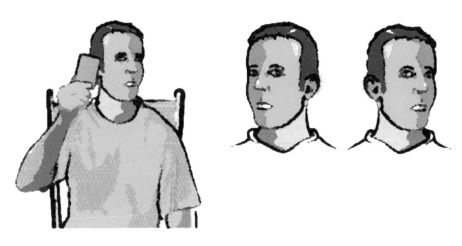

CHAPTER 3

OCULAR MOTOR EXERCISES

SMOOTH PURSUIT/TRACKING

Patients should be given this exercise when their ENG pursuit test shows ANY abnormalities. This can include significantly increased or decreased gain, saccadic intrusions, inverted pursuit, square wave pursuit, or any subjective patient complaints of dizziness or lightheadedness while performing the testing. This exercise should also be given if the patient has subjective complaints with any type of eye movements utilizing the pursuit reflex, even if not symptomatic during the testing.

Generally, it is best to start patients sitting and tracking in just the horizontal and vertical directions, 15 to 20 repeats in each direction. Progress by moving the patient to standing (feet apart, feet together, feet pointed), faster eye movements, increased number of repeats, diagonal plane movements, and/or lowered lighting. Also, progress patients by having them move the target card to a busy visual background, such as a checkerboard.

(Target cards and checkerboard are available in the Appendix section.)

SMOOTH PURSUIT/TRACKING

1) This exercise is to be performed _____ repeats.

2) This exercise is to be performed in the:
   ❑ horizontal plane
   ❑ vertical plane
   ❑ diagonal plane

3) This exercise is to be performed:
   ❑ eyes open
   ❑ eyes closed

4) This exercise is to be performed:
   ❑ sitting, supported
   ❑ sitting, unsupported
   ❑ standing, supported and ❑ feet shoulder-width apart ❑ feet together
   ❑ standing, unsupported and ❑ feet shoulder-width apart ❑ feet together
   ❑ standing on a foam cushion

5) Hold the target card 12-18 inches in front of your eyes. Be sure you can focus on the letters on the card.

6) Slowly move the card back and forth (horizontally), left and right in front of your eyes. Change hands, if necessary, to keep the card in view at all times. Keep your head still and focus on the letters of the card, moving only your eyes. DO NOT MOVE THE CARD SO FAST THAT THE LETTERS BECOME BLURRED OR OUT OF FOCUS!

7) Progress by moving in the vertical plane and/or the diagonal plane. Progress by placing the target card in the center of a busy visual background, such as a checkerboard. All progressions should be directed by your therapist. Try to keep increasing the speed at which you move the card. Remember to keep the letters on the card in focus and to move only your eyes with the card, not your head.

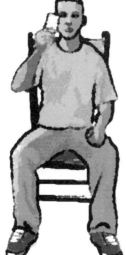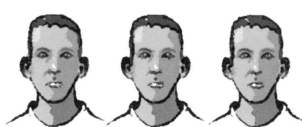

Remember: Move only your eyes.

SACCADE EYE MOVEMENTS

Patients should be given this exercise when their ENG saccade testing shows ANY abnormalities. This can include decreased velocity, increased latency, inaccuracy in any form, asymmetry, over- or undershoots, glissades, dysmetria of any sort, or any subjective patient complaints of dizziness or lightheadedness while performing the testing. This exercise should also be given if the patient has subjective complaints with any type of eye movements utilizing the saccade reflex, even if not symptomatic during the testing.

Generally, it is best to start patients sitting and moving their eyes in just the horizontal and vertical directions, 15 to 20 repeats in each direction. Progress by moving the patient to standing (feet apart, feet together, feet pointed), faster eye movements, increased number of repeats, diagonal plane movements, and/or lowered lighting.

SACCADE EYE MOVEMENTS

1) This exercise is to be performed _____ repeats.

2) This exercise is to be performed in the:
   ❑ horizontal plane
   ❑ vertical plane
   ❑ diagonal plane

3) This exercise is to be performed:
   ❑ eyes open
   ❑ eyes closed

4) This exercise is to be performed:
   ❑ sitting, supported
   ❑ sitting, unsupported
   ❑ standing, supported and   ❑ feet shoulder-width apart   ❑ feet together
   ❑ standing, unsupported and   ❑ feet shoulder-width apart   ❑ feet together
   ❑ standing on a foam cushion

5) Hold the target card 12-18 inches in front of your eyes. Be sure you can focus on the letters on the card.

6) Keeping the cards *and* your head still, moving only your eyes, jump your eyes back and forth between the two cards. Take about one second per card and find a specific letter on which to focus on each card. Spell out words or sentences to vary the exercise.

7) Progress by moving the cards into the vertical plane and/or the diagonal plane as directed by your therapist. Try to keep increasing the speed at which your eyes are moving. Remember to keep the letters on each card in focus and use only your eyes, not your head, to move from one target card to the other.

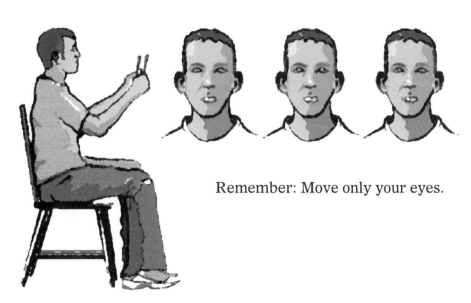

Remember: Move only your eyes.

OPTOKINETIC EYE MOVEMENTS

Patients should be given this exercise when their ENG Optokinetic (OpK) testing shows ANY abnormalities. This can include decreased speed (slow phase velocity), asymmetry, or any subjective patient complaints of dizziness or lightheadedness while performing the testing. This exercise should also be given if the patient has subjective complaints with any type of eye movements utilizing the optokinetic reflex, even if not symptomatic during the testing.

Generally, it is best to start patients sitting and moving their eyes in just the horizontal and vertical directions, 15 to 20 repeats in each direction. Progress by moving to patient standing (feet apart, feet together, feet pointed), faster eye movements, increased number of repeats, diagonal plane movements, and/or lowered lighting.

An OpK generator (black & white striped paper) is located in the Appendix.

OPTOKINETIC EYE MOVEMENTS

1) This exercise is to be performed _____ repeats.

2) This exercise is to be performed in the:
   ❑ horizontal plane
   ❑ vertical plane
   ❑ diagonal plane

3) This exercise is to be performed:
   ❑ eyes open
   ❑ eyes closed

4) This exercise is to be performed:
   ❑ sitting, supported
   ❑ sitting, unsupported
   ❑ standing, supported and ❑ feet shoulder-width apart ❑ feet together
   ❑ standing, unsupported and ❑ feet shoulder-width apart ❑ feet together
   ❑ standing on a foam cushion

5) Hold the optokinetic generator 12-18 inches in front of your eyes. Be sure you can focus on the letters on the card.

6) Keeping your head still, move the target slowly in front of your eyes, focusing on the center of the target.

7) Progress by moving the target into the vertical plane and/or the diagonal plane as directed by your therapist. Try to keep increasing the speed at which the target is moving. Remember to keep your head still. Have a partner look at your eye movements while doing the exercise. They should be "jumping" back and forth—a nystagmus movement.

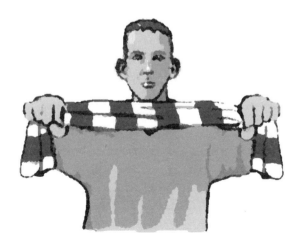

44

EXAMPLES OF EYE MOVEMENTS
FOR OCULAR MOTOR EXERCISES

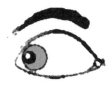 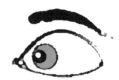 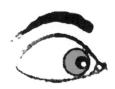 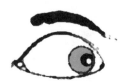

SIDE / SIDE

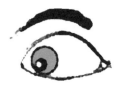 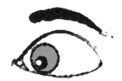 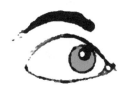 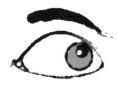

DIAGONALLY

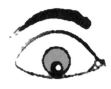 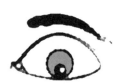 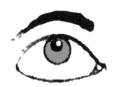 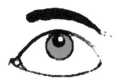

UP / DOWN

CHAPTER 4

BENIGN PAROXYSMAL POSITIONAL VERTIGO (BPPV)

BENIGN PAROXYSMAL POSITIONAL VERTIGO

Benign paroxysmal positional vertigo, with an incidence estimated at 600 cases per 100,000 population, is the most common balance disorder of the vestibular system. An estimated 20% of all patients with dizziness symptoms have this disorder. First described by Barany in 1921, the posterior canal variant is most prevalent; however, it can also occur in the superior and horizontal semicircular canals. The vertical canal variation can be induced by the classic headhanging (Dix-Hallpike) position and is characterized by:

- a horizontal or torsional, usually geotropic nystagmus;
- nystagmus associated with a subjective vertigo sensation; the nystagmus may reverse direction when the patient is moved back to the sitting position;
- a latency of several seconds between the assumption of the provoking position and onset of symptoms;
- a decrease in symptoms within 60 seconds of assuming the provoking position;
- and fatigability (i.e., a decrease in symptoms with repeated provocation).

BPPV involving either the posterior or superior canal (the vertical canals) is treated with the Particle Repositioning Maneuver.

The much rarer form involving the horizontal semi-circular canal is characterized by pure horizontal nystagmus when the patient is lying supine with the head either flat or slightly (<30 degrees) elevated. Again, there is a subjective vertigo sensation experienced by the patient while the nystagmus is visualized. There is also latency, short duration of symptoms and fatigablity. Patients with horizontal canal BPPV are treated with the "Bar-be-que Roll" maneuver.

Clinical observation of these signs and symptoms has led to the formulation of two commonly accepted theories of etiology: cupulolithiasis and canalithiasis. Common to both theories is the concept of otoconial crystal debris making the semicircular canals gravity sensitive. Cupulolithiasis, first described by Schuknecht (1969), postulates that otoconial debris from the utricle attaches to the cupula, changing its density relative to that of the surrounding endolymph. As a result, this structure becomes sensitive to the effects of gravity. When the patient's head is then placed in the provoking position, the cupula is deflected and vertigo results. Patients with this variant frequently have little latency to onset of symptoms and longer-lasting nystagmus and vertigo.

The second theory, canalithiasis, (Hall et al. 1979) postulates that otoconial debris does not attach to the cupula, but rather is free-floating within the semi-circular canal itself. The debris is sensitive to the effects of gravity and migrates to the most gravity-dependent position of the head. Movement of the particles within the canal results in displacement of the endolymphatic fluid, thereby causing a deflection of the cupula, resulting in nystagmus and vertigo.

Currently both etiologies are believed to exist, with canalithiasis by far the more common. Based on these theories of the mechanism of BPPV, numerous treatment strategies have been described and the literature contains many studies comparing the efficacy of these various procedures (Epley 1992; Girardi 1996; Herdman 1990; Semont 1988). The two broad categories of treatment are vestibular rehabilitation exercises and particle repositioning maneuvers. Vestibular rehabilitation exercises work on the premise that the CNS can be trained or "habituated" to the effects of vertigo. The repositioning maneuvers, on the other hand, were created to move debris out of the semi-circular canals and into the vestibule, using the effects of gravity and change in head position to relocate the otoconial crystals into the vestibule. The lining of the vestibule contains a number of enzymatic cells, called "dark cells," which have the function of creating and breaking down the calcium carbonate otoconial crystals.

The Particle Repositioning Maneuver (PRM) is performed on patients diagnosed with posterior or superior canal BPPV. The patient is placed in the provoking side Dix/Hallpike position (affected ear down) for three minutes following the cessation of symptoms. (Shake or roll the head if nystagmus or symptoms are not induced. If symptoms of torsional nystagmus—usually accompanied by vertigo—are not elicited, do not continue.)

The patient's head is then slowly turned (10-15 seconds) to the opposite D/H position (affected ear up), where it is maintained for an additional three minutes. Then the patient is rolled onto his/her shoulder, with the head facing downward to floor, and is kept in this position for an additional one minute. With the head supported, the patient is slowly returned to sitting position while the head is slowly rotated to facing front. If nystagmus is visualized and vertigo experienced by the patient after he/she has been moved to the sitting position, the entire procedure should be repeated. Frequently, patients will complain of lightheadedness or mild disequilibrium after assuming the sitting position. This is a common occurrence caused by orthostatic blood pressure changes and has no significance regarding the possible efficacy of the treatment.

Patients are given written instructions not to move their head and not to lie down flat for 24-48 hours following treatment. Also they should be told not to lie on the affected side for five days following that initial 24-48 hour period. Patients may be given a soft cervical collar to wear for the initial 24-48 hours to assist them in restricting their head movements.

Patients are then seen for follow-up of efficacy of treatment 7-14 days after the maneuver was performed. Treatment is performed without the patient meeting all six criteria for BPPV, but symptoms must be positionally provoked and include the characteristic nystagmus. Treatment is performed on patients with any etiology for the symptoms as well as for those patients with idiopathic BPPV (Girardi 1992).

Patients with a horizontal canal BPPV are treated utilizing the "Bar-be-que Roll" maneuver. They are maintained in each head position for one minute. The patient is first moved to the supine position, head turned toward the direction of the affected ear so the "bad" ear is down. After one minute, the head is rotated so the nose points upward. After one minute, the head is rotated another 90 degrees so the affected ear is now up and the "good" ear is down. After one minute, the patient is flipped from supine (lying on his/her back) to prone (lying on his/her stomach) with the nose pointed straight down to the floor. Assistance from a second therapist may be required for patient movement.

Following one minute, the patient's head is rotated another 90 degrees so that the affected ear is now down. After one minute, the patient is moved from prone, back to supine, with the nose facing straight up. After one minute, the patient is assisted to the sitting position, fitted with a soft cervical collar, and given the standard instructions of no head movements for 24-48 hours, including not lying down flat to sleep (Herdman 1994).

Lately, many vestibular laboratories have been combining habituation exercises with PRM treatments in an attempt to cure and/or prolong the remission of BPPV and have shown anecdotally that a combined approach may be more effective. A controlled study (Amin et al. 1999) yielded data that quantify the length of remission comparing particle repositioning alone with particle repositioning and vestibular rehabilitation. This project was designed to determine the efficacy of performance of the Brandt-Daroff (1980) habituation exercises following a successful Particle Repositioning Maneuver (PRM) to prolong the BPPV patients' remission and/or prevent the recurrence of their symptoms.

The results of this study indicate that the Brandt-Daroff exercises performed after a successful PRM prevented the recurrence of symptoms when compared to control subjects who performed no exercises. It was hypothesized that daily performance of exercises prevented the re-accumulation of debris in amounts significant enough to affect the cupula. Without cupular deflection, symptoms are not evident. If this is indeed the case, those individuals in whom otoconial degeneration is secondary to age or trauma would probably benefit from the performance of the exercises, as these persons would be most likely to experience unprovoked recurrences resulting from dislocation of otoconial debris. Individuals in whom BPPV was brought about by Meniere's disease or a viral infection may not find the post-maneuver exercises as beneficial.

Unlike the daily spontaneous dislocation of the otoconia that may occur with trauma or age, BPPV episodes triggered by Meniere's disease or labyrinthitis are more likely the result of discrete, single episodes. Therefore, the gradual build-up of particles in the posterior semi-circular canal seen with trauma or age would not be seen with Meniere's disease or labyrinthitis. However, it is recommended that all patients with BPPV who have been successfully treated with any single-treatment maneuver be instructed in the daily performance of the Brandt-Daroff exercises. The protocol calls for three repeats in each direction, done once daily.

REFERENCES

Amin, M., M. Girardi, M.A. Neill, L.F. Hughes, and H.R. Konrad. 1999. Effects of exercise on the prevention of recurrence of BPPV symptoms. Presented at the ARO Midwinter Meeting, St. Petersburg Beach, FL. Abstract published in the Abstracts of the 1999 ARO Midwinter Meeting.

Barany, R. 1921. Diagnose von krankheisterscheinungen im bereiche des otolinthenapparatus. *Acta Oto-Laryngol* 2:434.

Brandt, T., and R.B. Daroff. 1980. Physical therapy for benign paroxysmal positional vertigo. *Arch Otolaryngol* 6:484-85.

Dix, R. and C.S. Hallpike. 1952. The pathology, symptomology and diagnosis of certain common disorders of the vestibular system. *Proc. R. Soc. Med.* 45:341-54.

Epley, J.M. 1992. The canalith repositioning procedure for treatment of benign paroxysmal positional vertigo. *J. Otol. Head Neck Surg.* 107:399-404.

Girardi, M., and H.R. Konrad. 1996. Management of benign paroxysmal positional vertigo, *ORL Head and Neck Nursing* 4:25-30.

Hall, S.F., R.R.F. Ruby, and J.A. McLure. 1979. The mechanisms of benign paroxysmal vertigo. *J. Otolaryngol* 8:151.

Herdman, S.J. 1990. Treatment of benign paroxysmal positional vertigo. *Physical Therapy* 70:381-88.

Herdman, S.J., ed. 1994. Assessment and management of BPPV. In *Vestsibular rehabilitation*, 331-46. Philadelphia, F.A. Davis.

Semont, A., G. Freyess, and E. Vitte. 1988. Curing the BPPV with a liberatory maneuver. *Adv. Oto-Rhino-Laryngol* 42:290-93.

Schuknecht, H.F. 1969. Cupuliolithiasis. *Arch. Otolaryngol* 90:765.

THE PARTICLE REPOSITIONING MANEUVER (PRM) FOR TREATMENT OF POSTERIOR AND SUPERIOR CANAL BPPV

1) From a sitting position, turn the patient's head about 45 degrees toward the affected ear (in this illustration, the left). If this head turn provokes vertigo and/or nystagmus, do not continue with the treatment.

2) Quickly move the patient to the provoking side Dix/Hallpike position. Assess for nystagmus and vertigo. If you do not elicit a response, slightly shake or roll the head. If symptoms are not forthcoming, do not continue with the procedure. If symptoms of nystagmus and vertigo are provoked, allow the patient's head to remain in the Dix/Hallpike position for an additional three minutes after the cessation of symptoms.

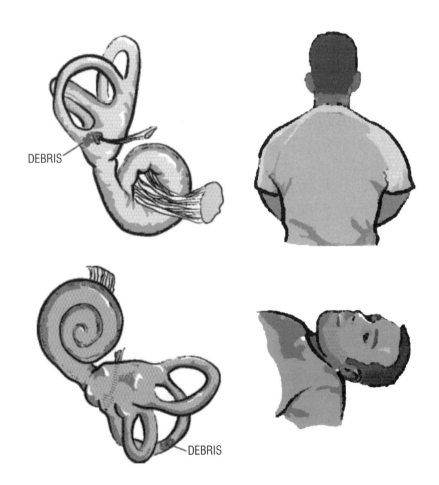

DEBRIS

DEBRIS

BRANDT-DAROFF EXERCISES—
TO PREVENT THE RECURRENCE OF BPPV

If you develop neck or back pain, or if your position-provoked vertigo returns for more than a few seconds, stop doing the exercise and contact our office immediately.

1) Sit on the side of your bed with your feet flat on the floor.

2) Turn your head to the left, looking up toward the ceiling.

3) As rapidly as possible, fall to the right side, resting on your right shoulder. Turn your head slightly upward.

4) Stay in this position for as long as your symptoms last (or for 10-15 seconds if you do not have symptoms of vertigo or dizziness).

5) Sit up as rapidly as possible, pushing up with your left arm. Then turn your head to the right and fall down onto your left shoulder. Keep your head facing slightly upward.

6) Stay in this position for as long as your symptoms last (or for 10-15 seconds if you do not have symptoms of vertigo or dizziness).

7) Alternating sides, repeat the exercise a total of three times in both directions.

8) Do this exercise once daily.

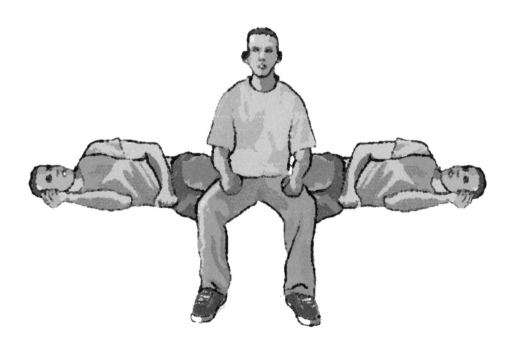

THE "BAR-BE-QUE ROLL" MANEUVER
FOR HORIZONTAL CANAL BPPV

Maintain each head position for one minute.

1) The patient is first moved to the supine position, head turned toward the direction of the affected ear so the "bad" ear is down (in this illustration, the left ear).

2) After one minute, the head is rotated so the nose points upward.

3) After one minute, the head is rotated another 90 degrees so the affected ear is now up and the "good" ear down.

4) After one minute, the patient is flipped from supine (lying on his/her back) to prone (lying on his/her stomach) with the nose pointed straight down to the floor. Assistance from a second therapist may be required for patient movement.

5) Following one minute, the patient's head is rotated another 45 degrees so that the affected ear is now down again.

6) After one minute, the patient is moved from prone back to supine, with the nose facing straight up.

7) After one minute, the patient is assisted to the sitting position, fitted with a soft cervical collar, and given the standard instructions of no head movements for the next 48 hours, and not lying flat to sleep.

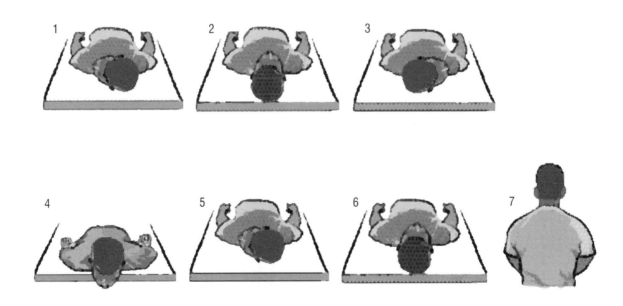

53

CHAPTER 5

EXERCISES TO IMPROVE BALANCE

GAZE STABILIZATION WHILE STANDING ON A COMPLIANT SURFACE

Patients should be given this exercise when their ENG gaze evoked or spontaneous nystagmus tests show ANY abnormalities. Generally, this means gaze evoked and/or spontaneous nystagmus of any type: horizontal, vertical, torsional, or oblique that is present and recorded as well as visualized. This can also include any subjective patient complaints of dizziness or lightheadedness while performing the testing. If the caloric test shows a failure of fixation suppression or if there are abnormalities on the auto-rotational VOR testing test, this exercise should be given. This exercise should also be given if the patient has subjective complaints with any type of eye or head movements, even if not symptomatic during the testing. This exercise would be added after the patient can successfully perform gaze stabilization while sitting and then standing.

Lastly, if the results of the patient's CAPS™ or other posturography tests show any type of balance deficits, this exercise should be used.

Generally, it is best to start patients standing with feet shoulder-width apart and moving their heads in just the horizontal and vertical directions, 15 to 20 repeats in each direction. Progress by moving patient to other stances (feet together, feet pointed), faster head movements, increased number of repeats, diagonal plane movements, and/or lowered lighting. Also, progress patients by having them move the target card to a busy visual background, such as a checkerboard.

GAZE STABILIZATION WHILE STANDING ON A COMPLIANT SURFACE

1) This exercise is to be performed _____ repeats.

2) This exercise is to be performed in the:
   ❑ horizontal plane
   ❑ vertical plane
   ❑ diagonal plane

3) This exercise is to be performed:
   ❑ eyes open
   ❑ eyes closed

4) This exercise is to be performed:
   ❑ standing, unsupported and
   ❑ feet shoulder-width apart
   ❑ feet together

5) Hold the target card 12-18 inches in front of your eyes. Be sure you can focus on the letters on the card.

6) Keeping the card still and your eyes focused on the letters on the card, slowly move your head back and forth (horizontally), left and right. DO NOT MOVE YOUR HEAD SO FAST THAT THE LETTERS BECOME BLURRED OR OUT OF FOCUS!

7) Progress by moving your head in the vertical plane and/or the diagonal plane. Progress by placing the target card in the center of a busy visual background, such as a checkerboard. All progressions should be directed by your therapist. Try to keep increasing the speed that your head is moving. Remember to keep the letters on the card in focus—move only your head.

TOSSING AND CATCHING A BALL

Patients should be given this exercise when their auto-rotational VOR testing test shows ANY abnormalities. This can include significantly increased or decreased gain or phase or abnormal symmetry or any subjective patient complaints of dizziness or lightheadedness while performing the testing. This exercise should also be given if the patient has subjective complaints with any type of head and eye movements utilizing the pursuit reflex, even if not symptomatic during the testing.

Lastly, if the results of the patient's CAPS™ or other posturography tests show any type of balance deficits, this exercise should be used.

Generally, it is best to start patients sitting and tossing and catching the ball in the vertical direction, 15 to 20 repeats. Progress by having the patient bounce the ball off a surface approximately 6 feet away and then catch it. Further progress by moving patient to standing (feet apart, feet together, feet pointed), faster body movements, increased number of repeats. Also, progress patients by having them play "catch" with a partner. Be sure the patient incorporates both head and eye movements in the exercise, keeping his or her eyes focused on the ball at all times.

TOSSING AND CATCHING A BALL
(with or without a partner)

1) This exercise is to be performed____repeats.

2) This exercise is to be performed
   ❑ sitting, supported.
   ❑ sitting, unsupported.
   ❑ standing, supported and ❑ feet shoulder-width apart ❑ feet together
   ❑ standing, unsupported and ❑ feet shoulder-width apart ❑ feet together
   ❑ standing on a foam cushion.

3) Use a medium-sized ball for this exercise.
   (soccer ball, basketball, volleyball, etc.)

4) Keep your eyes fixed on the ball and move your head and eyes so that you are always looking at the ball.

5) Toss the ball into the air and catch it.

6) Bounce the ball off a wall at least 6 feet away and catch it.

7) Progress by moving from sitting to standing. Progress by moving to playing catch with someone else. Be sure to keep your eyes fixed on the ball at all times, using eye and head movements. All progressions should be directed by your therapist.

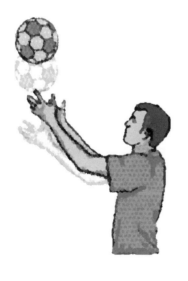

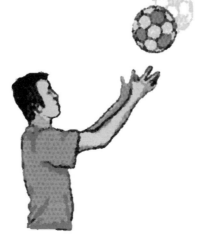

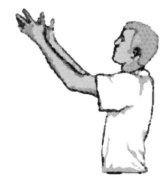

MOVING A BALL IN CIRCLES

Patients should be given this exercise when their auto-rotational VOR testing tests show ANY abnormalities. This can include significantly increased or decreased gain or phase or abnormal symmetry or any subjective patient complaints of dizziness or lightheadedness while performing the testing. This exercise should also be given if the patient has subjective complaints with any type of head and eye movements utilizing the pursuit reflex, even if not symptomatic during the testing.

Lastly, if the results of the patient's CAPS™ or other posturography tests show any type of balance deficits, this exercise should be used.

Generally, it is best to start patients sitting and moving a ball in a large circle. Progress by moving to standing with feet apart, then feet together, then pointed, and finally, standing on compliant foam.

Be sure the patient incorporates head and eye movements in the exercises, keeping his or her eyes focused on the ball at all times.

MOVING A BALL IN CIRCLES

1) This exercise is to be performed _____ repeats.

2) This exercise is to be performed:
   ❑ sitting, supported.
   ❑ sitting, unsupported.
   ❑ standing, supported and ❑ feet shoulder-width apart ❑ feet together.
   ❑ standing, unsupported and ❑ feet shoulder-width apart ❑ feet together.
   ❑ standing on a foam cushion.

3) Use a medium-sized ball for this exercise:
   soccer ball, basketball, volleyball, etc.

4) Keep your eyes fixed on the ball and move your head and eyes so that you are always looking at the ball.

5) Begin the exercise sitting. Move the ball in a large circle, over your head and down, almost sweeping the floor. Bend at the waist.

6) Progress by moving to a standing posture, feet shoulder-width apart. Again, make a big circle with the ball, moving your eyes and head so that you are always looking at the ball. Move the ball all the way over your head. Bend at the waist and the knees to move the ball downward, toward the floor. Progress by moving the ball faster and by narrowing your base of support by moving your feet closer together. All progressions should be directed by your therapist.

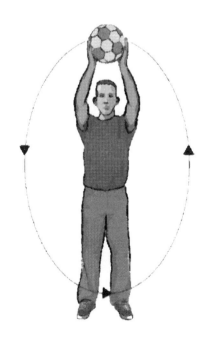

ANKLE SWAYS
(forward & back; left & right)

Patients should be given this exercise when they complain of imbalance, have a history of falling, or have any sort of disequilibrium when standing or walking. Also, if the results of the patient's CAPS™ or other posturography tests show any type of balance deficits, this exercise should be used.

Begin with the patient standing, feet shoulder-width apart for better stability. Progress the patient by narrowing the stance, moving eventually to standing on a perturbed surface. The patient is to sway, first forward and back, then side to side, moving only at the ankles. Also progress by having them hold the specific position for longer amounts of time. Begin with the patient having eyes open and focusing on a target on the wall. Another progression is to graduate to eyes closed, but have the patient imagine a target for a focal point.

Be careful to give this exercise only when the patient has demonstrated an ability to stand unsupported and is not at risk of falling.

ANKLE SWAYS
(forward & back; left & right)

1) This exercise is to be performed _____ repeats.

2) This exercise is to be performed moving:
❑ forward & backward
❑ left & right

3) This exercise is to be performed:
❑ sitting, supported
❑ sitting, unsupported
❑ standing, supported and ❑ feet shoulder-width apart ❑ feet together
❑ standing, unsupported and ❑ feet shoulder-width apart ❑ feet together
❑ standing on a foam cushion

4) This exercise is done standing with your eyes focused on a target on the wall, MOVING ONLY AT YOUR ANKLES. (DO NOT bend at the shoulders, waist, hips, or knees.) Sway your body forward as far as you can, moving your weight onto the balls of your feet. Do not let your heels come up off the floor! Do not move so much that you lose your balance and need to take a step. Hold the position for 5 seconds, then move back to standing straight upright. Wait 5 seconds, then repeat.

5) Then do the exercise by swaying your body backward, moving your weight over your heels. MOVE ONLY AT YOUR ANKLES! Do not let your toes come up off the floor. Do not move so much that you lose your balance and need to take a step. Hold the position for 5 seconds, then move back to standing straight upright. Wait 5 seconds, then repeat.

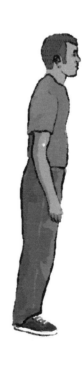

6) Sway to the left, moving your weight onto your left leg. Move as far as you can without your right leg coming off the floor. MOVE ONLY AT YOUR ANKLES! Do not move so much that you lose your balance and need to take a step. Hold the position for 5 seconds, then move back to standing straight upright. Wait 5 seconds, then repeat.

7) Sway to the right, moving your weight onto your right leg. Move as far as you can without your left leg coming off the floor. MOVE ONLY AT YOUR ANKLES! Do not move so much that you lose your balance and need to take a step. Hold the position for 5 seconds, then move back to standing straight upright. Wait 5 seconds, then repeat.

8) Progress by moving faster and by holding the leaning position for longer amounts of time. All progressions should be directed by your therapist.

ANKLE SWAYS
(circular)

Patients should be given this exercise when they complain of imbalance, have a history of falling, or have any sort of disequilibrium when standing or walking. Also, if the results of the patient's CAPS™ or other posturography tests show any type of balance deficits, this exercise should be used.

Have the patient sway in a circle, then step, then repeat in the opposite direction. Be certain that patients move in both the clockwise and counterclockwise directions.

Begin with the patient standing, feet shoulder-width apart for better stability. Progress the patient by narrowing the stance, moving eventually to standing on a perturbed surface. Also, progress by having them move faster. Begin with the patient having eyes open and focusing on a target on the wall. Another progression is to graduate to eyes closed, having the patients imagine a target for a focal point.

Be careful to give this exercise only when the patient has demonstrated an ability to stand unsupported and is not at risk of falling.

ANKLE SWAYS
(circular)

1) This exercise is to be performed _____ repeats.

2) This exercise is to be performed:
   ❑ sitting, supported
   ❑ sitting, unsupported
   ❑ standing, supported and ❑ feet shoulder-width apart ❑ feet together
   ❑ standing, unsupported and ❑ feet shoulder-width apart ❑ feet together
   ❑ standing on a foam cushion

3) This exercise is done standing with your eyes focused on a target on the wall. MOVING ONLY AT YOUR ANKLES (DO NOT bend at the shoulders, waist, hips, or knees), sway your body in a large circle by shifting your weight over your feet. KEEP BOTH FEET FLAT ON THE FLOOR. Do not move so much that you lose your balance and need to take a step. Perform the exercise in both the clockwise and counterclockwise directions.

4) Progress by moving more quickly and by increasing the number of times the exercise is repeated.

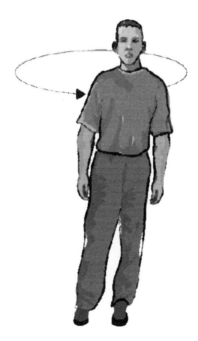

CHAPTER 6

EXERCISES
TO IMPROVE GAIT

SIDE STEPPING

Patients should be given this exercise when they complain of imbalance, have a history of falling, have any abnormalities of gait, or have any sort of disequilibrium when standing or walking. Lastly, if the results of the patient's CAPS™ or other posturography tests show any type of balance deficits, this exercise should be used.

Begin with the patient standing, feet together, ankles touching, and standing with his/her back against a flat wall for support. Have the patient move the left foot out, approximately 6-8 inches, then slide the right foot next to the left foot. Repeat several times. Then, reverse directions and move back the other direction, moving the right foot first, followed by the left. Progress the patient by increasing the speed at which the exercise is performed, by increasing the speed, and by moving away from the supporting wall. Lastly, when the patient becomes proficient, it can be performed with eyes closed.

Be careful to give this exercise only when the patient has demonstrated an ability to stand and move relatively unsupported and is not at risk of falling when performing the exercise.

SIDE STEPPING

1) This exercise is to be performed _____ repeats.

2) This exercise is to be performed:
   ❑ standing, supported by a wall behind you
   ❑ standing, unsupported

3) Stand with your back against a flat wall for support. Standing still, with your feet together, slide your left leg to the side about 6-8 inches. Then slide your right leg to the left so that both feet are touching. Repeat.

4) Then, repeat the process by sliding your right leg to the side about 6-8 inches. Then, slide your left leg to the right so that both feet are touching. Repeat.

5) Progress by moving your feet farther apart each time, by moving more rapidly and by moving away from the wall. All progressions should be directed by your therapist.

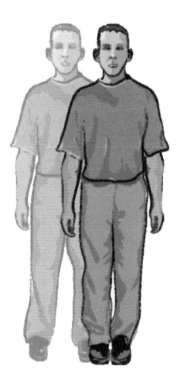

BODY ROLLING ALONG WALL

Patients should be given this exercise when they complain of imbalance, have a history of falling, have any abnormalities of gait, or have any sort of disequilibrium when standing or walking. Also, if the patient's CAPS™ or other posturography test results show any type of balance deficits, this exercise should be used.

Begin with the patient standing, feet shoulder-width apart, and pressing their back against a flat wall for support. Have the patient slowly move his/her feet, one at a time, so that the patient "rolls" his/her body along the wall. Repeat several times. Then, reverse directions and move back the other direction, rolling the body the opposite way.

Progress the patient by increasing the speed at which the exercise is performed, by increasing the speed, and by moving away from the supporting wall. Lastly, when the patient becomes proficient, it can be performed with eyes closed.

Be careful to give this exercise only when the patient has demonstrated an ability to stand and move relatively unsupported and is not at risk of falling when performing the exercise.

BODY ROLLING ALONG WALL

1) This exercise is to be performed _____ repeats.

2) This exercise is to be performed:
   ❑ standing, supported by a wall behind you.
   ❑ standing, unsupported.

3) This exercise is to be performed:
   ❑ eyes open.
   ❑ eyes closed.

4) Stand with your back against a flat wall for support. Slowly moving your feet, begin to turn your body and roll to the left, supported by the wall. Make one full 360 degree circle so that you end as you began, with your back to the wall.

5) Then, repeat the process but move in the opposite direction, rolling your body to the right, sliding your right leg to the side about 6-8 inches. Repeat the entire process.

6) Progress by moving your feet more rapidly and by moving away from the wall. Eventually, do the exercise with your back to the wall, but with your eyes closed. All progressions should be directed by your therapist.

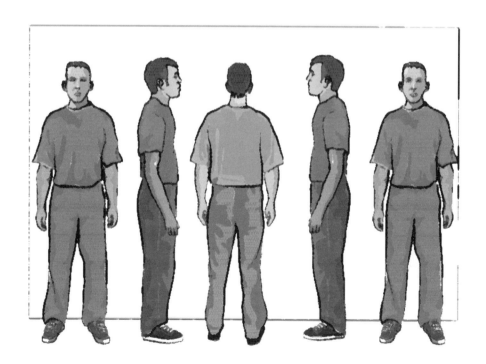

CROSS-OVER STEPPING

Patients should be given this exercise when they complain of imbalance, have a history of falling, have any abnormalities of gait, or have any sort of disequilibrium when standing or walking. Also, if the patient's CAPS™ or other posturography test results show any type of balance deficits, this exercise should be used.

Begin with the patient standing, feet shoulder-width apart, and standing with his/her back against a flat wall for support. Have the patient move the right foot, crossing it over and in front of the left foot. Then, the left foot is moved behind the right so that the patient is again standing with feet shoulder-width apart. This should be repeated several times. Then, have the patient reverse directions by moving the left foot, crossing it over and in front of the right foot.

Progress the patient by increasing the speed at which the exercise is performed, by increasing the amount of spread between the feet when crossing over, by starting with feet together (ankles touching), and by moving away from the supporting wall. Lastly, when the patient becomes proficient, it can be performed with eyes closed.

Be careful to give this exercise only when the patient has demonstrated an ability to stand and move relatively unsupported and is not at risk of falling when performing the exercise.

CROSS-OVER STEPPING

1) This exercise is to be performed _____ repeats.

2) This exercise is to be performed:
   ❑ standing, supported by a wall behind you.
   ❑ standing, unsupported.

3) Stand with your back against a flat wall for support. Standing still, with your feet shoulder-width apart, move your right leg in front of your left, crossing over. Then, move your left leg behind the right, so that you are again standing with feet shoulder-width apart. Repeat.

4) Repeat the process by moving your left leg crossing in front of the right. Go back to the "feet shoulder-width apart stance" by moving the left leg behind the right. Repeat.

5) Progress by moving your feet farther apart each time, by moving more rapidly by starting from a stance with feet together and ankles touching, and by moving away from the wall. All progressions should be directed by your therapist.

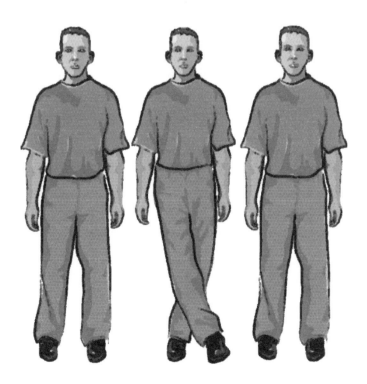

72

GAZE STABILIZATION WHILE WALKING

Patients should be given this exercise when their ENG gaze-evoked or spontaneous nystagmus tests show ANY abnormalities. Generally, this means gaze-evoked and/or spontaneous nystagmus of any type—horizontal, vertical, torsional, or oblique—that is present and recorded, as well as visualized. This can also include any subjective patient complaints of dizziness or lightheadedness while performing the testing. This exercise should also be given if the patient has subjective complaints with any type of eye or head movements, even if not symptomatic during the testing. This exercise should be added after the patient can successfully perform gaze stabilization while sitting and then standing.

Patients should be given this exercise when they complain of imbalance, have a history of falling, have any abnormalities of gait, or have any sort of disequilibrium when standing or walking. Also, if the patient's CAPS™ or other posturography test results show any type of balance deficits, this exercise should be used.

Generally, it is best to start patients standing with feet shoulder-width apart with a clear area of at least 10 feet in front of them. A hallway is an excellent place to perform this exercise. Patients begin walking forward and with every second step, a head turn is made. The head should be turned opposite the supporting foot: if the left foot is forward, the head turn is to the right; if the right foot is forward, the head is turned to the left. Repeat several times.

The exercise should be repeated with head movements in the vertical plane (up and down) as well. At all times, patients should attempt to walk as straight a line as possible, not veering left or right. Have them repeat several times. Progress patients by having them walk faster and move their heads faster, and by lowering the lighting in the room. Be careful to give this exercise only when the patient has demonstrated an ability to stand and move relatively unsupported and is not at risk of falling while performing the exercise.

GAZE STABILIZATION WHILE WALKING

1) This exercise is to be performed _____ repeats.

2) With your eyes focused on a target directly in front of you, walk at least 10 feet toward the target. Try to walk as straight as you can, not veering left or right, but keeping your eyes fixed on the target. Repeat.

3) Progress by walking faster and by lowering the room lighting. Also, progress by placing the target in the center of a busy visual background, such as a checkerboard. All progressions should be directed by your therapist. Remember to keep the target in focus as you walk.

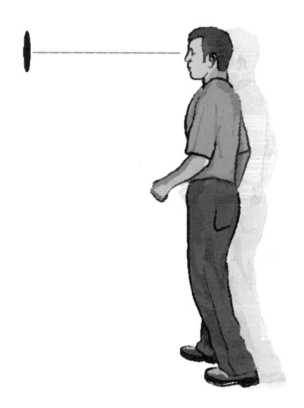

WALKING WITH HEAD MOVEMENTS

Patients should be given this exercise when their ENG gaze-evoked or spontaneous nystagmus tests show ANY abnormalities. Generally, this means gaze-evoked and/or spontaneous nystagmus of any type—horizontal, vertical, torsional, or oblique—that is present and recorded, as well as visualized. This can also include any subjective patient complaints of dizziness or lightheadedness while performing the testing.

This exercise should also be given if the patient has subjective complaints with any type of eye or head movements, even if not symptomatic during the testing. This exercise would be added after the patient can successfully perform gaze stabilization while sitting and then standing, then walking with head still.

Patients should be given this exercise when they complain of imbalance, have a history of falling, have any abnormalities of gait, or have any sort of disequilibrium when standing or walking. This exercise should also be used if the patient's CAPS™ or other posturography test results show any type of balance deficits.

Generally, it is best to start patients standing with feet shoulder-width apart and focusing on a target at least 10 feet in front of them. With their eyes fixed on the target, they begin walking toward it, trying to keep their gait as normal as possible. Then every other step, they should turn their head back and forth, left and right. They should also attempt to walk as straight a line as possible, not veering left or right. Have them repeat several times. Progress patients by lowering the lighting in the room, by having them make more rapid head movements, by having them do vertical head movements (up and down), and by having them walk faster.

WALKING WITH HEAD MOVEMENTS

1) This exercise is to be performed _____ repeats.

2) This exercise is to be performed with head movements:
   ❑ in the horizontal plane.
   ❑ in the vertical plane.

3) Standing at the end of a hallway or an open area at least 10 feet long, begin walking. With every other step, move your head left and right: when your right foot is forward, move your head to the left; when your left foot is forward, move your head to the right. Try to walk as straight as you can, not veering left or right, but keeping your eyes fixed on the target. Repeat.

4) Progress by moving your head in the vertical direction, looking up or down every other step.

5) Progress by walking faster, by moving your head faster, and by lowering the room lighting. All progressions should be directed by your therapist.

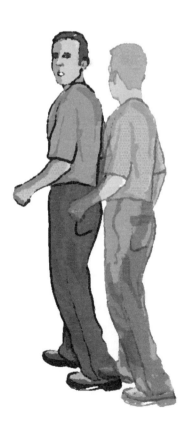

WALKING WITH QUICK STOPS

Patients should be given this exercise when they complain of imbalance, have a history of falling, have any abnormalities of gait, or have any sort of disequilibrium when standing or walking. Also, if the patient's CAPS™ or other posturography test results show any type of balance deficits, this exercise should be used.

Generally, it is best to start patients standing with feet shoulder-width apart and focusing on a target at least 10 feet in front of them. With eyes fixed on the target, they begin walking toward it, trying to keep their gait as normal as possible. They should also attempt to walk as straight a line as possible, not veering left or right. After a few steps, they should stop abruptly, trying to maintain their balance by correct use of ankle strategies. Have them repeat several times. Progress patients by having a partner call out the word "stop" when they are not expecting it, at which point the patient should stop. Other progressions include lowering the lighting in the room, walking faster, and eventually walking with the head in motion in both the vertical and horizontal planes before stopping abruptly.

WALKING WITH QUICK STOPS

1) This exercise is to be performed _____ repeats.

2) This exercise is to be performed with:
   ❑ head movements in the horizontal plane
   ❑ head movements in the vertical plane
   ❑ no head movements—looking straight ahead

3) Standing at the end of a hallway or an open area at least 10 feet long, begin walking. Look at a target at the end of the hallway. After a few steps, stop abruptly. Use sway around your ankles to remain in balance and upright. Start walking again. Repeat.

4) Progress by having someone tell you when to stop when you are not expecting it. Progress by moving your head left and right. Progress by moving your head in the vertical direction, looking up or down every other step.

5) Progress by walking faster, by moving your head faster, and by lowering the room lighting. All progressions should be directed by your therapist.

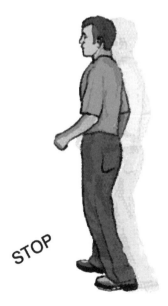

STOP

WALKING WITH QUICK STOPS & TURNS

Patients should be given this exercise when they complain of imbalance, have a history of falling, have any abnormalities of gait, or have any sort of disequilibrium when standing or walking. Also, if the patient's CAPS™ or other posturography test results show any type of balance deficits, this exercise should be used.

Generally, it is best to start patients standing with feet shoulder-width apart and focusing on a target at least 10 feet in front of them. With eyes fixed on the target, they begin walking toward it, trying to keep their gait as normal as possible. They should also attempt to walk as straight a line as possible, not veering left or right. After a few steps, they should stop abruptly, trying to maintain balance by correct use of ankle strategies. Once they are certain of their balance at the stop, they should quickly turn 180 degrees (facing the opposite direction) and begin walking again as soon as possible. Have them repeat several times, being certain to turn both left and right.

Progress patients by having a partner call out the word "stop" when they are not expecting it, at which point they stop. The partner then says "left" or "right" and the patient turns in the direction indicated. A further progression is to turn a full 360 degrees, then continue walking. Again, they should be instructed to turn both to the left and the right. Other progressions include lowering the lighting in the room, walking faster, and eventually walking with the head in motion in both the vertical and horizontal planes before stopping quickly and making the turns.

WALKING WITH QUICK STOPS & TURNS

1) This exercise is to be performed ____ repeats.

2) This exercise is to be performed with:
   ❑ head movements in the horizontal plane.
   ❑ head movements in the vertical plane.
   ❑ no head movements—looking straight ahead.

3) Standing at the end of a hallway or an open area at least 10 feet long, begin walking. Look at a target at the end of the hallway. After a few steps, stop abruptly. Use sway around your ankles to remain in balance and upright. Immediately turn around 180 degrees to the left, so you are now facing opposite the direction in which you began. Start walking again and repeat, this time turning to the right. Repeat each direction.

4) Progress by having someone tell you to stop when you are not expecting it. Your partner should then tell you "left" or "right" and you should turn in that direction. Progress by moving your head left and right. Progress by moving your head in the vertical direction, looking up or down every other step. Progress by turning a full 360 degree circle so you end up facing the same direction in which you started. Be careful to regain your full balance after you stop, before you begin to turn.

5) Progress by walking faster, by moving your head faster, and by lowering the room lighting. All progressions should be directed by your therapist.

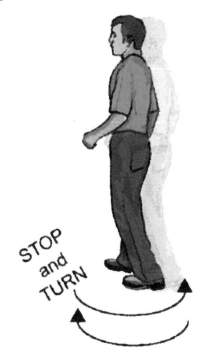

STOP and TURN

TANDEM WALKING

Patients should be given this exercise when they complain of imbalance, have a history of falling, have any abnormalities of gait, or have any sort of disequilibrium when standing or walking. Also, if the patient's CAPS™ or other posturography test results show any type of balance deficits, this exercise should be used. Patients should have successfully progressed through all other walking exercises before starting this one.

Generally, it is best to start patients standing with feet shoulder-width apart and focusing on a target at least 10 feet in front of them. With eyes fixed on the target, they begin walking toward it, trying to keep their gait as normal as possible. The patient should walk by placing one foot directly in front of the other, as though walking a tightrope. They should also attempt to walk as straight a line as possible, not veering left or right.

Patients should begin with arms extended outward to improve balance and progress to arms at the sides, eventually progressing to arms folded in front of them. Other progressions include lowering the lighting in the room; walking faster; eventually, walking with the head in motion in both the vertical and horizontal planes; and lastly, stopping quickly, then rapidly continuing the tandem gait.

TANDEM WALKING

1) This exercise is to be performed ____ repeats.

2) This exercise is to be performed with:
    ❑ no head movements—looking straight ahead
    ❑ head movements in the horizontal plane
    ❑ head movements in the vertical plane

3) This exercise is to be performed with arms:
    ❑ stretched outward
    ❑ at your side
    ❑ folded across your chest

4) Standing at the end of a hallway or an open area at least 10 feet long, begin walking. Look at a target at the end of the hallway. Walk by placing one foot directly in front of the other, as though you were walking on a tightrope. Repeat.

5) Progress by moving your arms first to your sides and eventually folded across your chest in front of you.

6) Progress by moving your head left and right. Progress by moving your head in the vertical direction, looking up or down every other step.

7) Progress by walking faster, by moving your head faster, by stopping abruptly and restarting to walk, and by lowering the room lighting. All progressions should be directed by your therapist.

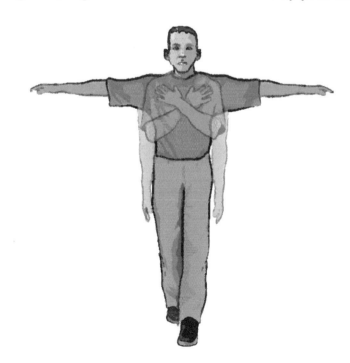

CHAPTER 7

MAINTENANCE EXERCISES

EXERCISE: LONG-TERM MAINTENANCE

When patients have successfully completed a VRT program, either home-based or in-house, they should be given a long-term maintenance exercise therapy program. After achieving the maximum level of compensation, without stimulation of the various inputs to balance, decompensation can occur. Therefore, patients should be given an exercise routine consisting of eye, head, and body movements to be performed daily, for at least 10-15 minutes. Some excellent long-term maintenance exercises are progressive walking with head movements and eye movements. This can be done in the home, out of doors, at a mall, or gym situation. Another suggestion is enrollment in a Tai Chi program. A third option is a custom-designed obstacle course.

EXERCISE: OBSTACLE COURSE

This exercise can be customized for any patient, based on his/her level of compensation, home/work environment, and physical abilities. Use your imagination to make the obstacle course as interesting and challenging as possible in order for the patient to compliantly perform the exercise. Utilize any items that may be readily at hand in the home or work environment. Try to match the various parts of the exercise with specific complaints the patient had at their original visit and any deficits seen during the ENG, CAPS™, or other posturography testing.

This specific example involves a chair, a box, a stool, and a ball. The patient is asked to sit in the chair and stand up several times. Other uses could be to sit and bend over, to walk around the chair several times in each direction before sitting and standing, etc. The patient could also be asked to perform ocular motor exercises while sitting.

The patient is then told to step over the box. Other uses could be to bend over, pick up the box, and lift it overhead; to pick up the box and turn 360 degrees before replacing it on the floor; or to pick up the box and place it on a shelf overhead, etc. These movements can be performed either with eyes open or eyes closed.

Next, the patient should go to the stool where he/she is asked to circle it several times in each direction. Other uses might be to sit down on the stool and stand up; to pick up the stool and move it several feet before sitting down and standing; and to tandem walk around the stool, etc. Lastly, the patient reaches the ball, at which point he/she is asked to pick up the ball and move it in a large circle, from overhead to sweeping the floor, by bending at the waist and knees. They are told to use head-and-eye movements to keep their gaze fixated on the ball at all times. Other instructions might be to toss the ball in the air and catch it; to bounce it off the floor or a wall; and to play "catch" with a partner, etc.

OBSTACLE COURSE

1) This entire battery of exercises is to be performed once daily.

2) Walk to the chair, sit in the chair, and stand up _____ times. Progress by sitting and bending over, and by walking around the chair several times each direction before sitting and standing.

3) Proceed to the box and step over it _____ times. Progress by bending over and picking up the box, lifting it overhead, and by picking up the box and turning 360 degrees before replacing it on the floor.

4) Go to the stool and walk a circle around it _____ times each direction. Progress by sitting down on the stool and stand up after you walk around it each time, pick up the stool and move it several feet before sitting down and standing, and then tandem walk around the stool.

5) Lastly, pick up the ball and move it in a large circle, from overhead to sweeping the floor by bending at the waist and knees. Use head-and-eye movements to keep your gaze fixated on the ball at all times. Progress by tossing the ball in the air and catching it, bounce it off the floor or a wall, and play "catch" with a partner.

Remember, all progressions should be directed by your therapist.

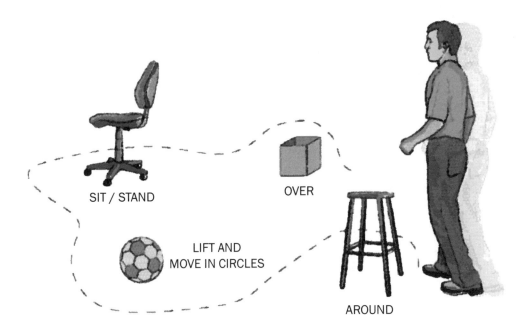

SIT / STAND   OVER

LIFT AND
MOVE IN CIRCLES

AROUND

APPENDIX

Give or mail to patients when an appointment for VRT is made.

VESTIBULAR REHABILITATION THERAPY PATIENT INFORMATION SHEET

You have been scheduled for a Dizziness and Balance Disorders Assessment in order to be treated with Vestibular Rehabilitation Therapy (VRT) for your dizziness/balance disorder.

The Clinic is located _____. Check in with the receptionist approximately 15 minutes before your scheduled appointment to complete necessary paperwork.

The assessment will take 30 to 90 minutes, and there is a slight chance that you may become somewhat dizzy, nauseated, or off-balance for a short time during or after the assessment. If possible, you should try to have someone accompany you to the first appointment and/or to be available to drive you home if necessary.

Our VRT is a specially tailored exercise program designed to improve your balance, lessen your dizziness, and help keep you from falling. It is performed as part of a home-based, self-motivated exercise program. You will be given specific exercises to perform in your home two to three times per day. We may wish to see you in the Clinic for additional therapy three or four times per week in the clinic. Generally, a VRT program will take approximately six to eight visits. Each follow-up visit will require about 30 minutes. If we feel it is necessary, you may be referred to other healthcare providers for additional services.

Assessment results and reports from subsequent visits will be sent to your referring physician, whom you may contact to discuss your ongoing care.

If you have questions regarding these instructions or if you require additional information about the testing, you may contact _____.

In order to obtain the most valid, highest quality results from the test and for your comfort and protection, please comply with the following instructions:

- **DO NOT DISCONTINUE MEDICATIONS FOR BLOOD PRESSURE CONTROL, CARDIAC OR CIRCULATORY PROBLEMS, DIABETES, THYROID, HORMONE REPLACEMENTS, OR ANY OTHER PRESCRIPTION MEDICATIONS UNLESS ADVISED TO DO SO BY YOUR PHYSICIAN!**

- If you have any questions regarding which medications may interfere with test results, please call the Clinic at _____ and/or contact your referring physician.

- **IF YOUR PHYSICIAN APPROVES, discontinue any anti-vertigo or vestibular suppressing medications for 48 hours prior to your appointment.** These include antivert, meclizine, bonine, dramamine, scopolomine, antihistimines, some sleeping pills, some pain medications, narcotics, or some tranquilizers (such as valium). Over-the-counter and prescription medications may adversely affect your therapy results.

- You may be asked to remove glasses/contact lenses prior to assessment.

- Wear loose comfortable clothing, preferably pants, and flat-heeled shoes for the assessment.

- If you must reschedule or cancel your appointment, please call the appointment desk **at least 24 hours prior** to your scheduled appointment time at _____.

90

90

Give or mail to patients when an appointment for CAPS™ is made.

CAPS™ PATIENT INFORMATION SHEET

You have been scheduled for a CAPS™ test, a computer-assisted evaluation of your sway, balance/stability, and risk of falling. In conjunction with that test, your vision and hearing may also be checked. The entire assessment will only take about 5 minutes.

The Clinic is located at _____.
Check in with the receptionist approximately 15 minutes before your scheduled appointment to complete necessary paperwork.

Test results will be sent to your referring physician who will discuss them with you and determine appropriate treatment strategies based on these (and other) results. If you have questions regarding these instructions or if you require additional information about the testing, please contact us. In order to obtain the most valid, highest quality test results and for your comfort and protection, please comply with the following instructions:

- **IF YOUR PHYSICIAN APPROVES, discontinue any anti-vertigo or vestibular suppressing medications for 48 hours prior to your appointment.** These include antivert, meclizine, bonine, dramamine, scopolomine, antihistimines, some sleeping pills, some pain medications, narcotics, or some tranquilizers (such as valium). Over-the-counter and prescription medications may adversely affect your therapy results. If you have any questions regarding which medications may interfere with test results, please call the Clinic at _____ and/or contact your referring physician.

- **DO NOT DISCONTINUE MEDICATIONS FOR BLOOD PRESSURE CONTROL, CARDIAC OR CIRCULATORY PROBLEMS, DIABETES, THYROID, HORMONE REPLACEMENTS, OR ANY OTHER PRESCRIPTION MEDICATIONS UNLESS ADVISED TO DO SO BY YOUR PHYSICIAN!**

- **Abstain from the use of excessive amounts of alcohol and caffeine (soft drinks/colas, coffee, tea, and chocolate) for 24 hours before the test.**

- For your vision test, please wear any glasses/contact lenses you normally wear. Wear loose comfortable clothing, preferably pants, and flat-heeled shoes for the test.

If you must reschedule or cancel your appointment, please call the appointment desk **at least 24 hours prior** to your scheduled appointment time at _____ .

Give or mail to patients when an appointment for CDP is made.

COMPUTERIZED DYNAMIC POSTUROGRAPHY
PATIENT INFORMATION SHEET

You have been scheduled for a Computerized Dynamic Posturography Assessment, which is a computer-assisted evaluation of the overall balance system for patients with dizziness, disequilibrium, or other balance disorders.

The Clinic is located at _____.
Check in with the receptionist approximately 15 minutes before your scheduled appointment to complete necessary paperwork.

The assessment will take 45 to 60 minutes, and there is a very slight chance that you may become somewhat dizzy, nauseated, or off-balance for a short time during or after the assessment. If possible, you should try to have someone accompany you to the first appointment and/or to be available to drive you home if necessary.

Test results will be sent to your referring physician who will discuss them with you and determine appropriate treatment strategies based on these (and other) results.

If you have questions regarding these instructions or if you require additional information about the testing, you may contact _____.

In order to obtain the most valid, highest quality results from the test and for your comfort and protection, please comply with the following instructions:

1. **IF YOUR PHYSICIAN APPROVES, discontinue any anti-vertigo or vestibular suppressing medications for 48 hours prior to your appointment.** These include antivert, meclizine, bonine, dramamine, scopolomine, antihistamines, some sleeping pills, some pain medications, narcotics, or some tranquilizers (such as valium). Over-the-counter and prescription medications may adversely affect your therapy results. If you have any questions regarding which medications may interfere with test results, please call the Clinic at _____ and/or contact your referring physician.

2. **DO NOT DISCONTINUE MEDICATIONS FOR BLOOD PRESSURE CONTROL, CARDIAC OR CIRCULATORY PROBLEMS, DIABETES, THYROID, HORMONE REPLACEMENTS, OR ANY OTHER PRESCRIPTION MEDICATIONS UNLESS ADVISED TO DO SO BY YOUR PHYSICIAN!**

3. **Abstain from the use of excessive amounts of alcohol and caffeine (soft drinks/colas, coffee, tea, and chocolate) for 24 hours before the test.**

4. You may be asked to remove glasses/contact lenses prior to assessment.

5. Wear loose comfortable clothing, preferably pants, and flat-heeled shoes for the assessment.

6. If you must reschedule or cancel your appointment, please call the appointment desk **at least 24 hours prior** to your scheduled appointment time at _____.

Give or mail to patients when an appointment for PRM is made.

PARTICLE REPOSITIONING MANEUVER (PRM) PATIENT INFORMATION SHEET

You have been scheduled for a Particle Repositioning Maneuver (PRM) for the treatment of Benign Paroxysmal Positional Vertigo (BPPV). This is a single treatment approach to resolve your vertigo symptoms. It has been shown to be highly effective.

The Clinic is located at _____.
Check in with the receptionist approximately 15 minutes before your scheduled appointment to complete necessary paperwork.

The therapy will take 30 to 45 minutes, and there is a slight chance that you may become somewhat dizzy or nauseated for a short time during or after the testing. Also, you will be asked to restrict your head movements for 48 hours after the treatment is performed. Therefore, you should try to have someone accompany you to the test and/or to be available to drive you home.

For the treatment, your head will be positioned in a fashion to move the debris particles causing your symptoms out of the semi-circular canals of the inner ear. You will be fitted with a soft cervical collar after treatment to assist in complying with the instructions of keeping your head still and not lying flat.

If you have questions regarding these instructions or if you require additional information about the testing, you may contact _____.

In order to obtain the most valid, highest quality results from the test and for your comfort and protection, please comply with the following instructions:

• **IF YOUR PHYSICIAN APPROVES, discontinue any anti-vertigo or vestibular suppressing medications for 48 hours prior to your appointment.** These include antivert, meclizine, bonine, dramamine, scopolomine, antihistamines, some sleeping pills, some pain medications, narcotics, or some tranquilizers (such as valium). Over-the-counter and prescription medications may adversely affect your therapy results. If you have any questions regarding which medications may interfere with test results, please call the Clinic at _____ and/or contact your referring physician.

1. **DO NOT DISCONTINUE MEDICATIONS FOR BLOOD PRESSURE CONTROL, CARDIAC OR CIRCULATORY PROBLEMS, DIABETES, THYROID, HORMONE REPLACEMENTS, OR ANY OTHER PRESCRIPTION MEDICATIONS UNLESS ADVISED TO DO SO BY YOUR PHYSICIAN!**

2. **Abstain from the use of excessive amounts of alcohol and caffeine (soft drinks/ colas, coffee, tea, and chocolate) for 24 hours before the test.**

3. You may be asked to remove glasses/contact lenses prior to treatment.

4. Wear loose comfortable clothing, preferably pants, and flat-heeled shoes for the treatment.

5. If you must reschedule or cancel your appointment, please call the appointment desk **at least 24 hours prior** to your scheduled appointment time at _____.

Give to patients immediately after performing PRM maneuver.

PATIENT INSTRUCTIONS FOLLOWING PARTICLE REPOSITIONING MANEUVER FOR BPPV

Following the treatment for your BPPV symptoms in the Clinic with the Modified Particle Repositioning Maneuver, you will be fitted with a soft cervical collar. We ask you to wear this collar for the 48 hours following the treatment, removing it only when absolutely necessary (bathing, changing clothing, etc.). When the collar is removed, be especially careful about not moving your head, particularly in the forward/backward plane. (Don't tilt your head back to rinse your hair or shave under your chin. Don't bend over with your head into the sink when brushing your teeth, etc.) For the entire 48-hour period, NO HEAD MOVEMENT IS PERMITTED! This includes turning the head left or right, looking up or down, bending over, etc. The more compliant you can be with these instructions, the more successful the outcome of your treatment is likely to be.

Also, for this 48-hour period, you may not lie down in the supine position (flat on your back), so sleeping must be done in a sitting up and slightly reclined position (head resting against the back of a soft chair, a pile of pillows, or one notch back in the recliner). Following the first 48 hours immediately after the treatment, you may remove the cervical collar. However, try to limit any very rapid head movements or head movements into the symptom-provoking position(s) for the next five days. During this five-day period, please refrain from sleeping with the treated ear down or with your head turned to the treated side, if possible.

You will need to return to the clinic 7 to 14 days following your initial treatment. Please schedule this important follow-up visit before you leave the clinic today. This visit is to determine how well the treatment worked for your problem. If you still have symptoms, another treatment may be performed or a different therapy utilized. If you are symptom-free at this point, you will be shown an exercise that has been shown to help prevent the return of your symptoms. If you have any questions regarding your treatment or these instructions, please contact one of the following individuals:

MENTAL STATUS EXAMINATION

Folstein, M.F., S.E. Folstein, and P.R. McHugh. 1975. Mini-mental state: A practical method for grading the cognitive states for the clinician. *J. Psychiatric Res.* 12:199-98.

Pfeiffer, E. 1975. Short portable mental status questionnaire. *J. Am. Geriatric Soc.* 23:433-41.

1. What is the date today? _____

2. What day of the week is it? _____

3. What is the name of this place? _____

4. What is your telephone number? _____

    Or alternatively, "What is your address?" _____

5. How old are you? _____

6. When were you born? _____

7. Who is the President of the United States now? _____

8. Who was the first President? _____

9. What was your mother's maiden name? _____

10. Subtract 3 from 20 and keep subtracting 3 from each new number, all the way down (20, 17, 14, 11, 8, 5, 2)

_____ Total number of errors

Scoring: 0-2 errors = oriented at all times
            3-4 errors = mild intellectual impairment
            5-7 errors = moderate intellectual impairment
            8-10 errors = severe intellectual impairment

VESTIBULAR REHABILITATION THERAPY (VRT)
PATIENT HISTORY & ASSESSMENT FORM

It is suggested that patients complete the intake survey and the DHI and bring the completed forms to the clinic on their first visit. Information can be briefly confirmed and condensed on this form during the patient contact time.

Name_____ Date_____

Address_____City, State, Zip_____

Home Phone_____ Work Phone _____

Date of birth _____ Age_____

Referring Physician_____

      Address_____

Other physician(s) to whom you want records sent _____

      Address_____

Name and phone number of relative/friend_____

HISTORY

Date of onset of symptoms: _____

Symptoms: _____

Duration: _____Causes:_____

Medical History: _____

Surgical History: _____

Medications: _____

Vision/Hearing: _____

ENG Results: _____

CDP Results: _____

History of Falls: _____

Description of Falls: _____

SUBJECTIVE

Home environment_____

Levels inside_____ Steps_____ Railings_____ Ramps_____

Assistive devices available_____

Assistance available_____

Social history_____

Past functional status_____

OBJECTIVE

General appearance _____

Posture_____

Cognitive status _____ ABC score _____ Mental Status Score_____

RANGE OF MOTION (ROM) AND MUSCLE STRENGTH

		Range of Motion		Strength	
		Left	Right	Left	Right
Upper Extremity					
Shoulder	Flexion	____	____	____	____
	Abduction	____	____	____	____
Elbow	Flexion	____	____	____	____
	Extension	____	____	____	____
Wrist	Flexion	____	____	____	____
	Extension	____	____	____	____
Finger	Flexion	____	____	____	____
	Extension	____	____	____	____
Lower Extremity					
Hip	Flexion	____	____	____	____
	Extension	____	____	____	____
Hip	Abduction	____	____	____	____
	Adduction	____	____	____	____
Knee	Flexion	____	____	____	____
	Extension	____	____	____	____
Ankle	Dorsi Flexion	____	____	____	____
	Plantar Flexion	____	____	____	____

WNL =within normal limits
WFL =within functional limits
N/A=not applicable/not assessed

5/5 = complete ROM against gravity with full resistance
4/5 = complete ROM against gravity with moderate resistance
3/5 = complete ROM against gravity
2/5 = complete ROM against gravity eliminated
1/5 = no contraction

PHYSICAL EXAM

Vital signs _____

Muscle Tone_____

Posturing, overflow_____ Increased resistance to passive stretch_____

Coordination_____

Finger to nose_____ Heel to shin_____

Finger tap_____ Toe/heel tap_____

Sensation_____

Pain Complaints_____

Deformities, contractures_____

VESTIBULAR FUNCTION TESTS

Spontaneous nystagmus
Gaze-evoked nystagmus
Center_____ Left_____ Right_____ Up_____ Down_____
Saccade
      Horizontal_____ Vertical_____
Pursuit
      Horizontal_____ Vertical_____
Optokinetic
      Horizontal_____ Vertical_____

Dix-Hallpike
Sitting head right_____ Supine head hanging right_____
Sitting head left_____ Supine head hanging left _____
Positional
      Shoulder right_____ Shoulder left_____
Other_____

Head movements/Still object_____

Head movements/Moving object in phase_____

Head movements/Moving object out of phase_____

Dynamic Visual Acuity_____

POSTURAL TESTS

Sitting: Passive/Active	Eyes Open	Eyes Closed

Anterior/Posterior

	Eyes Open	Eyes Closed
Weight shift	_____	_____
Head righting	_____	_____
Equilibrium reactions	_____	_____
Trunk recovers vertical	_____	_____
Dizziness	_____	_____
Protective response	_____	_____

Lateral

	Eyes Open	Eyes Closed
Weight shift	_____	_____
Head righting	_____	_____
Equilibrium reactions	_____	_____
Trunk recovers vertical	_____	_____
Dizziness	_____	_____
Protective response	_____	_____

Standing:
Alignment (symmetry and verticality) _____

Postural Movement	Strategy	Dizziness	Loss of Balance
Active: Anterior/Posterior	_____	_____	_____
Lateral	_____	_____	_____
Passive: Anterior/Posterior	_____	_____	_____
Lateral	_____	_____	_____

FUNCTIONAL TESTING

Chair Rising_____

Get Up and Go_____

Timed Up and Go_____

Romberg_____

Pointed Romberg_____

CTSIB_____

Functional Reach_____

Fukuda_____

Tinetti Balance_____

Tinetti Gait_____

Berg_____

Dynamic Gait_____

SUMMARY

Fall Factors

Cognitive_____

Sensory_____

Visual_____

Musculoskeletal_____

Coordination_____

Balance_____

Fall risk: Low   Mild   Moderate   High

Goals

Patient goals:_____

Immediate therapy goals	ACHIEVED	NOT ACHIEVED	N/A
1. Patient instructed on and issued a home exercise program	____	____	____
2. Patient demonstrated appropriate performance and understanding of home exercise program (a) independently, (b) with assistance of caregiver, (c) with future support of outpatient rehab services	____	____	____
3. Patient demonstrates appropriate compensatory strategies	____	____	____
4. Patient identifies fall risk factors	____	____	____
5. Other goals_____	____	____	____

Reason(s) for goal(s) not achieved: _____

Recommendations:

_____ Home-based exercises, follow-up with therapist

_____ Outpatient therapy (frequency) _____

_____ Home health therapy (frequency)_____

Rehabilitation potential: ___excellent ___good ___fair ___poor

PLAN

Treatment (type of exercise and frequency)

Patient/family education_____

BPPV Treatment_____

ROM exercises_____

Strengthening exercises_____

Ocular Motor exercises_____

Balance exercises_____

Gait exercises_____

Other_____

Therapist signature_____Date_____

Requirement for outpatients with Medicare:
I have reviewed this plan of care and certify that these services are medically necessary services.

Physician signature_____ Date_____

DIZZINESS HANDICAP INVENTORY

Jacobson, G.P., and C.W. Newman. 1990. The development of the dizziness handicap inventory. *Arch. Otolaryngol Head Neck Surg.* 116:424.

The purpose of this scale is to identify difficulties that you may be experiencing because of your dizziness or unsteadiness. Please answer "Yes," "No," or "Sometimes" to each question by writing the corresponding letter in the blanks on the right side of the paper. Answer each question as it pertains to your dizziness or unsteadiness only.

Y=Yes **S**=Sometimes **N**=No

P ⬚ 1) Does looking up increase your problem?

E ⬚ 2) Because of your problem, do you feel frustrated?

F ⬚ 3) Because of your problem, do you restrict travel for business and/or recreation?

P ⬚ 4) Does walking down the aisle of a supermarket increase your problem?

F ⬚ 5) Because of your problem, do you have difficulty getting into or out of bed?

F ⬚ 6) Does your problem significantly restrict your participation in social activities, such as going out to dinner, movies, dancing, or parties?

F ⬚ 7) Because of your problem, do you have difficulty reading?

P ⬚ 8) Does performing more ambitious activities like sports, dancing, and household chores, such as sweeping or putting dishes away, increase your problem?

E ⬚ 9) Because of your problem, are you afraid to leave your home without having someone accompany you?

E ⬚ 10) Because of your problem, have you been embarrassed in front of others?

P ⬚ 11) Do quick movements of your head increase your problem?

F ⬚ 12) Because of your problem, do you avoid heights?

P ⬚ 13) Does turning over in bed increase your problem?

F ⬚ 14) Does your problem make it hard for you to do strenuous house/yard work?

E ⬚ 15) Because of your problem, are you afraid people may think you are drunk?

F ⬚ 16) Because of your problem, is it difficult for you to go for a walk by yourself?

P ⬚ 17) Does walking down a sidewalk increase your problem?

E ⬚ 18) Because of your problem, is it difficult for you to concentrate?

F ⬚ 19) Because of your problem, is it difficult for you to walk around your house in the dark?

E ⬚ 20) Because of your problem, are you afraid to stay home alone?

E ⬚ 21) Because of your problem, do you feel handicapped?

E ⬚ 22) Has your problem placed stress on your relationships with members of your family or friends?

E ⬚ 23) Because of your problem, are you depressed?

F ⬚ 24) Does your problem interfere with your job or household responsibilities?

P ⬚ 25) Does bending over increase your problem?

FOR OFFICE USE ONLY: ❑ Initial visit ❑ Follow-up visit

F _____ (36) E _____ (36) P _____ (28) TOTAL _____ (100)

Scoring: 4 points for Yes; 2 points for Sometimes; 0 points for No.

Patient Name _____

ACTIVITIES-SPECIFIC BALANCE CONFIDENCE (ABC) SCALE

Powell, L.E., and A.M. Myers. 1995. The activities-specific balance confidence (ABC) scale. *J. Gerontol.: A Biol. Sci. Med. Sci.* 50A:M28-34.

Patients should be instructed to fill in one of the following percentages for each individual question. They should be told: "Even if you don't do this activity now, think about what your confidence level would be if you were performing the activity." They should answer 100% if they feel they would not lose their balance or become unsteady. If a task is usually performed with an aid, they should answer as if they were using the assistive device.

10%   20%   30%   40%   50%   60%   70%   80%   90%   100%
No confidence   **Complete confidence**

_____ 1. Walking around the house.

_____ 2. Walking up and down stairs inside the home.

_____ 3. Picking up a slipper or something from the floor.

_____ 4. Reaching at your eye level.

_____ 5. Reaching for something over your head while standing on your toes.

_____ 6. Reaching for something over your head while standing on a chair.

_____ 7. Sweeping the floor.

_____ 8. Walking outside to a nearby car.

_____ 9. Getting in or out of a car or other transportation.

_____ 10. Walking across a parking lot.

_____ 11. Walking up and down a ramp.

_____ 12. Walking in a crowded mall where people walk rapidly past you.

_____ 13. Being bumped while walking in a crowd.

_____ 14. Using an escalator while holding the railing.

_____ 15. Using an escalator while holding packages without holding the railing.

_____ 16. Walking on slippery floors or icy sidewalks.

Total Average Score _____ (<68% = low mobility, increased fear)

ROMBERG TEST &
SHARPENED/POINTED ROMBERG TEST

Black, F.O., C. Wall, H.F. Rocketter, et al. 1982. Normal subjects' postural sway during the Romberg test. *Am. J. Otolaryngol* 3:309-18.

The Romberg test is a traditional assessment of vestibule-spinal function but this is not a particularly sensitive test for instability, particularly for patients with a unilateral peripheral vestibular loss. It can be made more sensitive by modifying it to have the patient stand in the sharpened or pointed position (one foot directly behind the other). This classic test of quiet stance involves having the patient stand with feet together, arms crossed, and eyes closed. While it is easy to perform in most settings and can be quantified to a degree (amount of time patient can keep stance), it does not test the patient's adaptive response.

STANDING ON ONE LEG,
EYES OPEN AND EYES CLOSED
(SOLEO & SOLEC)

Heitmann, D.K., M.R. Gossman, S.R. Shaddeaus, et al. 1989. Balance performance and step width in non-instutionalized elderly female fallers and non-fallers. *Physical Therapy* 69:923-29.

While a more sensitive classical clinical assessment than the Romberg, this test can lack functional validity since many elderly and/or neurological patients may not be able to perform the tasks because of health issues that are unrelated to balance.

Patients are asked to stand on one leg with the knee flexed and the hips neutral and arms folded across the chest. First, they should be asked to perform the task with eyes open, then with eyes closed. They should be able to hold each stance for 30 seconds without putting the raised foot down, unfolding the arms, or opening the eyes. They should be given three attempts at each task.

FUKUDA STEPPING TEST

Fukuda, T. 1959. The stepping test: Two phases of the labyrinthine reflex. *Acta. Otolaryngol* 50:95.

Wantanabe, T., et al. 1985. Automated graphical analysis of Fukuda's stepping test. In *Vestibular and Visual Control on Posture and Locomotor Equilibrium*, eds. M. Igarashi, and F.O. Black, 80. Basel, Switzerland: Karger.

The Fukuda Stepping Test measures balance while the patient marches in place with eyes closed and arms outstretched forward at a 90-degree angle to the patient's body. The examiner should count silently 50 steps while closely guarding the patient to prevent a fall. Use a mark on the floor or a marked grid to note forward progression or rotation during the marching. Be certain to observe the direction and degree of rotational movement. Normal subjects move forward less than 50 centimeters and rotate less than 30 degrees at the end of the 50 steps. Patients with a unilateral peripheral deficit are highly likely to turn excessively, and usually in the direction of the side of lesion.

CLINICAL TEST OF SENSORY INTEGRATION IN BALANCE (CTSIB)

Horak, F.B. 1987. Clinical measurement of postural control in adults. *Physical Therapy* 67:1881-85.

Shumway-Cook, A., and F.B. Horak. 1986. Assessing the influence of sensory interaction on balance. *Physical Therapy* 66:1548-50.

This test can be performed if computer dynamic posturography is not available. Also referred to as the "foam and dome" test, this assessment looks at a patient's ability to integrate and use visual, vestibular, and somatosensory inputs under conditions where one or more sense is removed or perturbed. Originally, there were six sensory conditions: eyes open, firm surface; eyes closed, firm surface; eyes open, perturbed surface; eyes closed, perturbed surface; visual dome, firm surface; and visual dome, perturbed surface. Today, however, the visual dome conditions are usually not performed as it was found that there was little reliable variation between these conditions and the eyes closed conditions.

The foam should be a 16-inch by 18-inch, 2- to 3-inch thick T-foam. Patients should be able to perform each test under each condition for 30 seconds. They should be carefully guarded and observed for movement strategy (ankle, hip, step). There should be no foot or hand movements, and no conversation during the assessment.

While the test may indicate balance impairments and the ability to select appropriate sensory inputs, it is not as sensitive as the SOT test of computer dynamic posturography.

DYNAMIC GAIT INDEX

Shumway-Cook, A., and M. Woollacott. 1995. *Motor control: Theory and practical applications.* Baltimore: Williams and Wilkins.

Shumway-Cook A., et al. 1997. Predicting the probability for falls in the community-dwelling older adults. *Physical Therapy* 77:812.

This test is very useful in determining gait impairment in patients with vestibular and balance disorders.

Scoring: Mark each task with the lowest category which applies (4=best; 0=worst).

1. Gait on a level surface

  Instructions: Walk at your normal speed from the start to the next mark (20 feet).

  4=Normal: Walks 20 feet with no assistive devices, good speed, no evidence of imbalance, normal gait pattern.

  3=Mild impairment: Walks 20 feet, uses assistive device, slower speed, mild gait deviations.

  2=Moderate impairment: Walks 20 feet, slow speed, abnormal gait pattern, evidence of imbalance.

  1=Severe impairment: Cannot walk 20 feet without assistance, severe gait deviation or imbalance. _ _ _ _ _ _ _ _ _ _ _ _ _ ____

2. Change in gait speed

  Instructions: Begin walking at your normal pace for 5 feet. When I say "go," walk as fast as you can for 5 feet. When I tell you "slow," walk as slowly as you can for 5 feet.

  4=Normal: Able to smoothly change walking speed without loss of balance or gait deviation. Shows a significant difference in walking speeds between normal, fast, and slow speeds.

  3=Mild impairment: Is able to change speed but demonstrates mild gait deviations or no gait deviations, but unable to achieve a significant change in velocity or uses an assistive device.

  2=Moderate impairment: Makes only minor adjustments to walking speed, or accomplishes a change in speed with significant gait deviations, or changes speed but loses significant gait deviations, or changes speed but loses balance but is able to recover and continue walking.

  1=Severe impairment: Cannot change speeds, or loses balance and has to reach for wall or be caught. _ _ _ _ _ _ _ _ _ _ _ ____

108

3. Gait with horizontal head turns

Instructions: Begin walking at your normal pace. When I tell you to "look right," keep walking straight but turn your head to the right. Keep looking to the right until I tell you "look left," then keep walking straight and turn your head to the left. Keep your head to the left until I tell you "look straight," then keep walking straight but turn your head back to the center.

4=Normal: Performs head turns smoothly with no change of gait.

3=Mild impairment: Performs task with slight change in gait velocity, i.e., minor disruption to smooth gait path or uses walking aide.

2=Moderate impairment: Performs head turns with moderate change in gait velocity, slows down, staggers but recovers and can continue to walk.

1=Severe impairment: Performs task with severe disruption of gait, i.e., staggers outside 15-inch path, loses balance, stops, reaches for wall. _____ ____

4. Gait with vertical head turns

Instructions: Begin walking at your normal pace. When I tell you to "look up," keep walking straight, but tip your head and look up. Keep looking up until I tell you "look down," then keep walking straight and turn your head down. Keep looking down until I tell you "look straight," then keep walking straight and turn your head back to the center.

4=Normal: Performs head turns with no change in gait.

3=Mild impairment: Performs task with slight change in gait velocity, i.e., minor disruption to smooth gait path or uses walking aid.

2=Moderate impairment: Performs task with moderate change in gait velocity, slows down, staggers but recovers and can continue to walk.

1=Severe impairment: Performs task with severe disruption of gait, i.e., staggers outside 15-inch path, loses balance, stops, reaches for wall. _____ ____

5. Gait with pivot turns

Instructions: Begin walking at your normal pace. When I tell you to "turn and stop," turn as quickly as you can to face the opposite direction and stop.

4=Normal: Pivot returns safely within 3 seconds and stops quickly with no loss of balance.

3=Mild impairment: Pivot turns safely in >3 seconds and stops with no loss of balance.

2=Moderate impairment: Turns slowly, requires verbal cueing, requires several small steps to catch balance following turn and stop.

1=Severe impairment: Cannot turn safely, requires assistance to turn and stop. _____ ____

6. Step over obstacles

Instructions: Begin walking at your normal speed. When you come to the
shoebox, step over it, not around it, and keep walking.

4=Normal: Is able to step over box without changing gait speed; no
evidence for imbalance.

3=Mild impairment: Is able to step over box, but must slow down and
adjust steps to clear box safely.

2=Moderate impairment: Is able to step over box, but must stop, then step
over. May require verbal cueing.

1=Severe impairment: Cannot perform without assistance. _ _ _ _   _____

7. Step around obstacles

Instructions: Begin walking at your normal speed. When you come to the
first cone (about 6 feet away), walk around to the right side of it.
When you come to the second cone (6 feet past first cone,) walk
around it to the left.

4=Normal: Is able to walk around cones safely without changing gait
speed; no evidence of imbalance.

3=Mild impairment: Is able to step around both cones, but must slow
down and adjust steps to clear cones.

2=Moderate impairment: Is able to clear cones but must significantly
slow speed to accomplish task, or requires verbal cueing.

1=Severe impairment: Unable to clear cones, walks into one
or both cones, or requires physical assistance. _ _ _ _ _ _ _ _   _____

8. Stairs

Instructions: Walk up these stairs as you would at home (i.e., using the rail
if necessary). At the top, turn around and walk down.

4=Normal: Alternates feet, no use of rail.

3=Mild impairment: Alternates feet, must use rail for support.

2=Moderate impairment: Two feet to a stair,
must use rail for support.

1=Severe impairment: Cannot perform safely. _ _ _ _ _ _ _ _ _ _ _ _   _____

TOTAL SCORE: _____

BERG FUNCTIONAL BALANCE SCALE

Berg, K.O., S.L. Wood-Dauphine, J.L. Williams, et al. 1989. Measuring balance in the elderly: Development of an instrument. *Physiotherapy Canada* 41:304-11.

Berg, K.O., S.L. Wood-Dauphine, J.L. Williams, et al. 1992. Measuring balance in the elderly: Validation of an instrument. *Can. J. Public Health* Suppl. no. 2, 83:S7-11.

This test incorporates several other tests, such as Chair Rising, Get Up and Go, Functional Reach, Romberg, SOLEO, horizontal head movements, and stair climbing.

Scoring: Mark the lowest category which applies for each task (4=best, 0=worst).

1. Sitting to standing
> *Instruction: Stand up without using your hands for support.*
> 4=able to stand without hands and stabilize independently.
> 3=able to stand independently with use of hands.
> 2=after several tries, able to stand with use of hands.
> 1=needs minimal assistance to stand or to stabilize.
> 0=needs moderate or maximal assistance to stand. _ _ _ _ _ _ _ _ _   _ _ _ _

2. Standing unsupported
> Instruction: Stand safely for two minutes without holding onto anything.
> 4=able to stand safely for 2 minutes.
> 3=able to stand for 2 minutes with supervision.
> 2=able to stand for 30 seconds unsupported.
> 1=needs several tries to stand for 30 seconds unsupported.
> 0=unable to stand for 30 seconds unassisted. _ _ _ _ _ _ _ _ _ _ _ _ _   _ _ _ _

IF THE SUBJECT IS ABLE TO STAND SAFELY FOR 2 MINUTES, SCORE FULL MARKS (4) FOR SITTING UNSUPPORTED, THEN SKIP TASK #3 AND PROCEED TO TASK #4, "STANDING TO SITTING."

3. Sitting unsupported, feet flat on the floor
> *Instruction: Sit with arms folded for two minutes.*
> 4=able to sit safely for 2 minutes.
> 3=able to sit for 2 minutes with supervision.
> 2=able to sit for 30 seconds unsupported.
> 1=needs several tries to sit for 30 seconds unsupported.
> 0=unable to sit for 30 seconds unassisted. _ _ _ _ _ _ _ _ _ _ _ _ _   _ _ _ _

4. Standing to sit

Instruction: Sit down without using your hands.

4=sits safely with minimal use of hands.

3=controls descent by using hands.

2=uses back of legs against chair to control descent.

1=sits independently but has uncontrolled descent.

0=needs assistance to sit. _____ _____

5. Transfers

Instruction: Move from chair to bed and back again. Perform exercise
once using a chair with armrests and once using a chair without
armrests.

4=able to transfer safely with only minor use of hands.

3=able to transfer safely with definite need of hands.

2=able to transfer with verbal cueing and/or supervision.

1=needs one person to assist.

0=needs two people to assist and/or supervise to be safe. _____ _____

6. Standing unsupported with eyes closed

Instructions: Close your eyes and stand still for 10 seconds unsupported.

4=able to stand for 10 seconds safely.

3=able to stand for 10 seconds with supervision.

2=able to stand for 3 seconds.

1=unable to keep eyes closed for 3 seconds but stays steady.

0=needs help to keep from falling. _____ _____

7. Standing unsupported with feet together

Instruction: Place your feet together and stand unsupported.

4=able to place feet together independently and to stand
for 1 minute safely.

3=able to place feet together independently and to stand
for 1 minute with supervision.

2=able to place feet together independently but unable to hold stance
for 30 seconds.

1=needs help to attain position but able to stand
for 15 seconds with feet together.

0=needs help to attain position and unable to hold
for 15 seconds _____ _____

THE FOLLOWING TASKS ARE TO BE PERFORMED WHILE STANDING UNSUPPORTED:

8. Reaching forward with outstretched arm

> Instructions: Lift your arm and reach forward at a 90-degree angle to the floor. Stretch out your fingers and reach forward as far as you can, but do not move your feet. (Examiner places a ruler at the end of the fingertips before the patient begins reaching forward. The patient's fingers should not touch the ruler while reaching forward. The recorded measure is the distance forward that the fingers reach while the subject is in the most forward position.

4=can reach forward confidently >10 inches.

3=can reach forward >5 inches safely.

2=can reach forward >2 inches safely.

1=reaches forward but needs supervision.

0=needs help to keep from falling. _____ _____

9. Pick up an object from the floor

Instructions: Pick up an object that has been placed in front of your feet.

4=able to pick up object safely and easily.

3=able to pick up object but needs supervision.

2=unable to pick up but reaches 1-2 inches from object and keeps balance independently.

1=unable to pick up object and needs supervision while trying.

0=unable to try; needs assistance to keep from falling. _____ _____

10. Turning to look behind/over left and right shoulders

Instructions: Turn to look behind you over your left shoulder, then repeat to the right.

4=looks behind from both sides and weight shifts well.

3=looks behind one side only; other side shows less weight shift.

2=turns sideways only but maintains balance.

1=needs supervision when turning.

0=unable to try turning head;
needs assistance to keep from falling. _____ _____

11. Turning around 360 degrees

Instructions: Turn completely around in a full circle. Pause. Then turn a full circle in the other direction.

4=able to turn 360 degrees safely in <4 seconds for each side.

3=able to turn 360 degrees safely one side only in <4 seconds.

2=able to turn 360 degrees safely but slowly.

1=needs close supervision or verbal cueing to turn.

0=needs assistance to keep from falling;
unable to attempt turning. _____ _____

DYNAMIC WEIGHT SHIFTING WHILE STANDING UNSUPPORTED

12. Stepping up on a stool

Instructions: Place each foot alternately on the stool. Continue until each
foot has touched the stool four times.

4=able to stand independently and safely, and complete 8 steps
in 20 seconds.

3=able to stand independently and complete 8 steps in >20 seconds.

2=able to complete 4 steps without aid with supervision.

1=able to complete >2 steps but needs minimal assistance.

0=needs assistance to keep from falling;
unable to attempt steps. _____ ____

13. Standing unsupported, one foot in front of the other (tandem stance)

Instructions: (Examiner should demonstrate to subject.) Place one foot
directly in front of the other. If you feel that you cannot place one
foot directly in front, try to step far enough ahead that the heel of
your forward foot is ahead of the toes of the other foot.

4=able to place feet in tandem stance independently and hold stance for
30 seconds.

3=able to place feet in tandem stance independently and hold stance for
<30 seconds.

2=able to take a small step independently and hold stance for 30 seconds.

1=needs help to get into stance but can hold 15 seconds.

0=loses balance while getting into stance or while standing. ___ ____

14. Standing on one leg

Instructions: Stand on one leg as long as you can without holding onto
anything.

4=able to lift leg independently and hold one-legged stance for >10
seconds.

3=able to lift leg independently and hold one-legged stance for 5-10
seconds.

2=able to lift leg independently and hold on to support for >3 seconds.

1=tries to lift leg; unable to hold stance 3 seconds but remains standing
independently.

0=unable to attempt or needs assistance to prevent falling. ____ ____

TOTAL SCORE: ____ / **56**

Score >45 = Safe ambulation, without an assistive device/less likely to fall.
Score >35 = Safe ambulation with an assistive device.

ADAPTED TINETTI'S BALANCE
AND MOBILITY ASSESSMENT

Tinetti, M.E. 1986. Performance oriented assessment of mobility problems in elderly patients. *J. Am. Geriatr. Soc.* 34:119-26.

Tinetti, M.E., and S.F. Ginter. 1991. Identifying mobility dysfunctions in elderly patients: Standard neuromuscular examination or direct assessment? *JAMA* 259:1190-93.

_____

I. BALANCE TESTS

Initial instructions: Subject is seated in a hard, armless chair. The following maneuvers are tested.

1. Sitting balance

Leans or slides in chair = 0

Sits steady, safe = 1 _____ ____

2. Attempts to arise

Unable without help = 0

Able, but requires more than one attempt = 1

Able to rise unassisted, one attempt = 2 _____ ____

3. Arises

Unable without help = 0

Able, but uses arms to help = 1

Able, without using arms = 2 _____ ____

4. Immediate standing balance (first 5 seconds after rising)

Unsteady (swaggers, move feet, trunk sways) = 0

Steady, but uses walker, cane, or other support = 1

Steady without walker, cane, or other support = 2 _____ ____

5. Standing balance

Unsteady = 0

Steady but wide stance (medial heels >4 inches apart)
     and/or uses support = 1

Narrow stance without support = 2 _____ ____

6. Nudged *(subject at a maximum stance position with feet as close together as possible, examiner pushes lightly on subject's sternum with palm of hand three times)*

Begins to fall = 0

Staggers, grabs examiner, catches self = 1

Steady = 2 _____ ____

7. Standing, eyes closed (*at maximum position, feet together*)
     Unsteady = 0
     Steady = 1 _   ____

8. Turning 360 degrees
     Discontinuous steps = 0
     Unsteady (grabs examiner, staggers) = 1
     Continuous, smooth = 2 _   ____

9. Sitting down
     Unsafe (misjudged distance, falls into chair) = 0
     Uses arms or not a smooth motion = 1
     Safe, smooth motion = 2 _   ____

BALANCE SCORE: ____ / 16
(A score below 11 is indicative of a fall.)

II. GAIT TESTS

Initial Instructions: Subject stands with the examiner, walks down hallway, or across room; first at usual pace, then back at rapid, but safe pace (utilizing usual walking aids).

10. Initiation of gait (immediately after told to go)
     Any hesitancy of multiple attempts to start = 0
     No hesitancy = 1 _   ____

11. Step length and height
       a. Right foot swing
     Does not pass left foot with step = 0
     Passes left stance foot = 1
     Right foot does not clear floor completely with step = 0
     Right foot completely clears floor = 1 _ _ _ _ _ _ _ _ _ _ _ _ _ _ _ _ _   ____
       b. Left foot swing
     Does not pass right stance foot with step = 0
     Passes right stance foot = 1
     Left foot does not clear floor completely with step = 0
     Left foot completely clears floor = 1 _ _ _ _ _ _ _ _ _ _ _ _ _ _ _ _ _   ____

12. Step symmetry
     Right and left step length not approximately equal = 0
     Right and left step appear approximately equal = 1 _ _ _ _ _ _ _ _   ____

13. Step continuity

Stopping or discontinuity between steps = 0

Steps appear continuous = 1 _____ ____

14. Path *(Estimated in relation to floor tiles, 12-inch diameter;*

observe excursion of one foot over about 10 feet of the course)

Marked deviation = 0

Mild to moderate deviation or uses walking aid = 1

Straight without walking aid = 2 _____ ____

15. Trunk

Marked sway or uses walking aid = 0

No sway but flexion of knees or back pain or spreads arms out while

walking = 1

No sway, no flexion, no use of arms,

and no use of walking aid = 2 _____ ____

16. Walking stance

Heels apart, wide base = 0

Heels almost touching while walking = 1 _____ ____

GAIT SCORE: ____ / 12

(A score below 8 is indicative of a fall.)

COMBINED BALANCE AND GAIT SCORE: ____ / 28

(A score below 20 is indicative of a fall.)

DUNCAN FUNCTIONAL REACH TEST

Duncan, P.W., D.K. Weiner, J. Chandler, and S. Studenski. 1990. Functional reach: A new clinical measure of balance. *J. Gerontol.* 45:M195.

Duncan, P.W., S. Studenski, J. Chandler, and B. Prescott. 1992. Functional reach: Predictive validity in a sample of elderly male veterans. *J. Gerontol.* 47:M93-8.

This is a single item test developed as a quick screen for balance problems in older adults. It looks at limits of stability in standing. During the initial research, a high functioning, low risk for falling group of veterans scored a mean of 12.14 inches. Functionally impaired, high risk of falling elderly patients had a mean score of 7.4 inches.

Patients should be asked to stand with feet apart with one arm raised to 90 degrees flexion. While keeping their feet still, subjects reach as far forward as they can while still maintaining their balance. The distance reached is measured from a ruler fastened to the wall and compared to age-matched norms. This test has established inter-rater reliability and has been shown to be highly predictive of falls among older adults.

Functional Reach Age-matched Norms:

Age	Men (Range in inches)	Women (Range in inches)
20 – 40 years	14.80 – 18.6	12.4 – 16.8
41 – 69 years	12.7 – 17.1	11.6 – 16.0
70 – 87 years	11.6 – 14.8	7.0 – 14.0

CHAIR RISING PERFORMANCE

Merrill, S., et al. 1997. Gender differences in the comparison of self-reported disability and performance measures. *J. of Gerontology* 52A:M19.

This is an excellent, simple, easy, and time-efficient clinical tool to assess falls risks. It is particularly useful when doing mass screenings.

Have the patient sit in a hard-backed chair, feet flat on the floor, and the patient's back not touching the back of the chair. Ask the person to rise out of chair without using his/her hands.

The test has been shown to have a predictive relationship of increased likelihood of falling:

1) If use of hands or other assistance is necessary to stand up.

2) If a single trial takes more than 2 seconds.

3) If five consecutive trials, repeated one immediately after another, take more than 18.5 seconds.

GET UP AND GO TEST

Mathias, S., U. Nayak, and B. Isaacs. 1986. Balance in elderly patients: The get up and go test. *Arch. Phys. Med. Rehabil.* 67:387-89.

This test was developed as a quick screening tool for detecting balance problems in elderly patients. The test requires that individuals stand up from a chair, walk three meters (ten feet), turn around, and return to the chair and sit. Performance is scored according to the following scale:

1	=	normal
2	=	very slightly abnormal
3	=	mildly abnormal
4	=	moderately abnormal
5	=	severely abnormal

An increased risk for falls was found among older adults who scored three or above on this test.

TIMED UP AND GO TEST

Podsiadlo, D., and S. Richardson. 1991. The timed up and go: A test of basic functional mobility for frail elderly persons. *J. Am. Geriatr. Soc.* 39:142-48.

The Timed Up and Go test modifies the original test by adding a timing component to performance. Neurologically intact elderly adults who were independent in balance and mobility skills were able to perform the test in less than 10 seconds. Adults who took more than 30 seconds to complete the test were dependent in most activities of daily living and mobility skills.

The test requires that individuals stand up from a chair, walk three meters (ten feet), turn around, and return to the chair and sit.

HOME SURVEY FOR FALL PREVENTION

Josephson, K.R., D.A. Fabacher, and L.Z. Rubenstein. 1991. Home safety and fall prevention. *Clinics in Geriatric Medicine* 7:707-31.

Throughout the home
____(–) Presence of throw rugs.
____(–) Presence of loose carpeting.
____(–) Slippery floors.
____(–) Thresholds on floors.
____(–) Lighting causes glare.
____(–) Unlighted pathways to bedroom and bathroom.

Kitchen
____(+) Easy access to commonly used dishes.
____(+) Avoid shelves above easy reach.
____(+) Use footstool with handrail or not at all.

Bathroom
____(+) Rubber bath mat.
____(+) Showerhead extender.
____(+) Use shower chair with back and nonskid tips.
____(+) Install grab bars in shower and tub and alongside toilet.
____(+) Obtain raised seat and arms for toilet.

Bedroom
____(–) Too low or high of a bed.
____(–) Too soft of a mattress.
____(–) No bedrails.
____(+) Bedside commode or urinal.
____(+) Safe pathway to bathroom.

Stairs and Hallways
____(+) Handrails are easy to grasp and very visible.
____(+) Markers on top and bottom of handrail.
____(+) Light switches at top and bottom of stairs.
____(+) Nonskid surfaces on stairs.
____(+) Stair edges marked.

Outdoors
____(–) Clutter near walkways.
____(–) Snow and ice on paths.
____(+) Presence of lights and handrails.
____(–) Pathways contain soft gravel or uneven surfaces.

Assistive Devices/Footwear
____(+) Educated on the use of any assistive device.
____(+) Good tips of canes and walkers.
____(+) Wheelchair brakes and footrests are in good condition.
____(+) Proper footwear, avoiding loose shoes or slippery soles.

OCULAR MOTOR TESTS

If ENG results are unavailable, perform these tests as an observational office exam.

Gaze & Spontaneous Nystagmus Testing

For gaze-evoked nystagmus testing, have the patient seated. Looking at the patient's eyes in a well-lighted situation, have the patient focus on a target (examiner's finger). While watching the patient's eyes for nystagmus, keep the eyes in each position for 20-30 seconds. If nystagmus is seen, question the patient about subjective sensations of vertigo or imbalance. The following five positions are used: straight forward; eyes 20 degrees left; eyes 20 degrees right; eyes 20 degrees up; and eyes 20 degrees down. Do not go too far in any direction as a false positive result from endpoint nystagmus could be the result.

For the spontaneous nystagmus, if Frenzel glasses or infrared goggles are available, place them on the patient. If not, lower the room light as much as possible, leaving just enough diffuse light so the patient's eye movements are visible. Using the same five-eye positions, again observe the eyes for nystagmus and question the patient regarding subjective symptoms.

Smooth Pursuit Testing

With the patient seated, ask him/her to follow a moving target (examiner's finger) back and forth (left and right) in a sinusoidal pattern at a frequency of about 0.5 Hz. Watch the patient's eyes to observe smooth sinusoidal movement without saccadic intrusions or delays at specific points.

Saccade Testing

With the patient seated, ask him/her to follow a target (examiner's fingers) randomly moving in the horizontal plane. Change target position about every 1-3 seconds and perform 10-15 different movements. Watch the patient's eyes to observe smooth rapid movements without "stairstepping" and over-shooting or under-shooting the target.

Optokinetic Testing

With the patient seated, move the optokinetic target generator (black-and-white striped paper) in front of the patient's eyes. Have the patient focus on the center of the target while you move it back and forth (left and right) at a frequency of about 1 Hz. Observe the patient's eyes for OPK generated nystagmus in both directions.

122

A B C D E F   A B C D E F
G H I J K L   G H I J K L
M N O P Q R   M N O P Q R
S T U V W X   S T U V W X
Y Z 1 2 3 4   Y Z 1 2 3 4
5 6 7 8 9 0   5 6 7 8 9 0

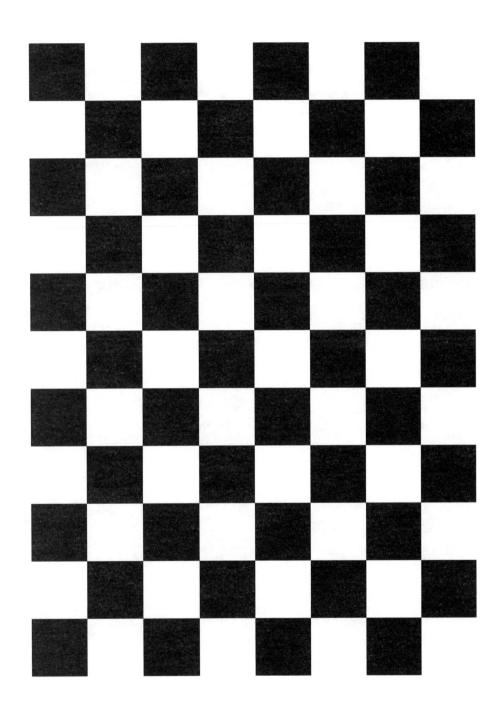

	Distance Equivalent
64	$\frac{20}{800}$
734	$\frac{20}{400}$
3986 ∃ ∃	$\frac{20}{200}$
5 2 3 7 Ш ∃ E ↑ → ↓	$\frac{20}{100}$
7 9 4 3 ∃ Ш E → ↑ ←	$\frac{20}{70}$
8 9 7 4 8 Ш E ∃ ← ↑ →	$\frac{20}{50}$
6 9 0 2 8 3 Ш ∃ Ш ↓ ↑ ↑	$\frac{20}{40}$
2 4 8 3 7 6 1 E Ш Ш ↓ ↓ ↓	$\frac{20}{30}$
9 2 7 8 6 5 8 4 Ш Ш E → ↑ ↑	$\frac{20}{25}$
8 9 9 4 0 3 7 2 E Ш Ш ← ↑ ↑	$\frac{20}{20}$

Hold card 14 inches from eyes with good lighting. Evaluate each eye individually and together, with or without glasses or bifocals.

Applications

od - right eye,   os - left eye,   ou - both eyes,   gtts-drops

Pupil Gauge (mm.)

2 3 4 5 6 7 8 9

REPRODUCIBLE
PATIENT HANDOUTS

The following 22 patient handouts may be freely copied and distributed to patients, as copyright has been waived on such materials.

GAZE STABILIZATION

1) This exercise is to be performed ____ repeats.

2) This exercise is to be performed in the:
   ❑ horizontal plane
   ❑ vertical plane
   ❑ diagonal plane

3) This exercise is to be performed:
   ❑ eyes open
   ❑ eyes closed

4) This exercise is to be performed:
   ❑ sitting, supported
   ❑ sitting, unsupported
   ❑ standing, supported and ❑ feet shoulder-width apart ❑ feet together
   ❑ standing, unsupported and ❑ feet shoulder-width apart ❑ feet together

5) Hold the target card 12-18 inches in front of your eyes. Be sure you can focus on the letters on the card.

6) Keeping the card still and your eyes focused on the letters on the card, slowly move your head back and forth (horizontally), left and right. DO NOT MOVE YOUR HEAD SO FAST THAT THE LETTERS BECOME BLURRED OR OUT OF FOCUS!

7) Progress by moving your head in the vertical plane and/or the diagonal plane. Progress by placing the target card in the center of a busy visual background, such as a checkerboard. All progressions should be directed by your therapist. Try to keep increasing the speed that your head is moving. Remember to keep the letters in the card in focus—move only your head.

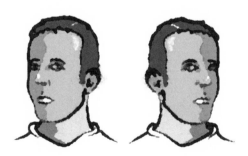

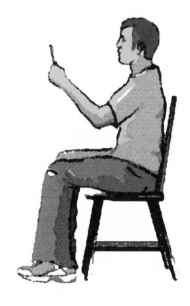

TIMES ONE VIEWING
Target In Phase with Head

1) This exercise is to be performed _____ repeats.

2) This exercise is to be performed in the:
   ❑ horizontal plane
   ❑ vertical plane
   ❑ diagonal plane

3) This exercise is to be performed:
   ❑ eyes open
   ❑ eyes closed

4) This exercise is to be performed:
   ❑ sitting, supported
   ❑ sitting, unsupported
   ❑ standing, supported and ❑ feet shoulder-width apart ❑ feet together
   ❑ standing, unsupported and ❑ feet shoulder-width apart ❑ feet together
   ❑ standing on a foam cushion

5) Hold the target card 12-18 inches in front of your eyes. Be sure you can focus on the letters on the card.

6) Slowly move the card left and right (horizontally), keeping your eyes focused on the letters on the target, and moving your entire upper body to go a full 180 degrees. Change hands, if necessary, to keep the card in view at all times. Move the entire upper body (not just your head) to maintain a focus on the letters of the card. DO NOT MOVE THE CARD AND YOUR HEAD SO FAST THAT THE LETTERS BECOME BLURRED OR OUT OF FOCUS!

7) Progress by moving in the vertical plane and/or the diagonal plane. Progress by placing the target card in the center of a busy visual background, such as a checkerboard. All progressions should be directed by your therapist. Try to keep increasing the speed at which the card and your head are moving. Remember to keep the letters in the card in focus and to use your entire upper body, not just your head, to move with the card.

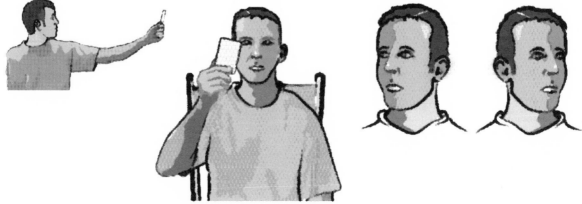

TIMES TWO VIEWING
Target Out of Phase with Head

1) This exercise is to be performed _____ repeats.

2) This exercise is to be performed in the:
   - ❏ horizontal plane
   - ❏ vertical plane
   - ❏ diagonal plane

3) This exercise is to be performed:
   - ❏ eyes open
   - ❏ eyes closed

4) This exercise is to be performed:
   - ❏ sitting, supported
   - ❏ sitting, unsupported
   - ❏ standing, supported and   ❏ feet shoulder-width apart   ❏ feet together
   - ❏ standing, unsupported and   ❏ feet shoulder-width apart   ❏ feet together
   - ❏ standing on a foam cushion

5) Hold the target card 12-18 inches in front of your eyes. Be sure you can focus on the letters on the card.

6) Slowly move the card left and right (horizontally), keeping your eyes focused on the letters on the target. Move your head in the opposite direction of the card movement. When the card is moved to the left, move your head to the right; when the card is moved to the right, move your head to the left; but make sure your eyes remain focused on the letters on the card at all times. DO NOT MOVE THE CARD OR YOUR HEAD SO FAST THAT THE LETTERS BECOME BLURRED OR OUT OF FOCUS!

7) Progress by moving in the vertical plane (target goes up, head goes down, eyes stay focused on the card, etc.) and/or the diagonal plane. Progress by placing the target card in the center of a busy visual background, such as a checkerboard. All progressions should be directed by your therapist. Try to keep increasing the speed at which you are moving both the card and your head, but remember to keep the letters on the card in focus at all times.

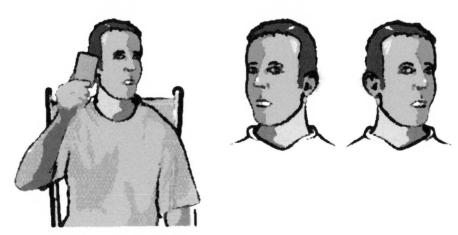

SMOOTH PURSUIT/TRACKING

1) This exercise is to be performed _____ repeats.

2) This exercise is to be performed in the:
   ❑ horizontal plane
   ❑ vertical plane
   ❑ diagonal plane

3) This exercise is to be performed:
   ❑ eyes open
   ❑ eyes closed

4) This exercise is to be performed:
   ❑ sitting, supported
   ❑ sitting, unsupported
   ❑ standing, supported and ❑ feet shoulder-width apart ❑ feet together
   ❑ standing, unsupported and ❑ feet shoulder-width apart ❑ feet together
   ❑ standing on a foam cushion

5) Hold the target card 12-18 inches in front of your eyes. Be sure you can focus on the letters on the card.

6) Slowly move the card back and forth (horizontally), left and right in front of your eyes. Change hands, if necessary, to keep the card in view at all times. Keep your head still and focus on the letters of the card, moving only your eyes. DO NOT MOVE THE CARD SO FAST THAT THE LETTERS BECOME BLURRED OR OUT OF FOCUS!

7) Progress by moving in the vertical plane and/or the diagonal plane. Progress by placing the target card in the center of a busy visual background, such as a checkerboard. All progressions should be directed by your therapist. Try to keep increasing the speed at which you move the card. Remember to keep the letters on the card in focus and to move only your eyes with the card, not your head.

Remember: Move only your eyes.

SACCADE EYE MOVEMENTS

1) This exercise is to be performed _____ repeats.

2) This exercise is to be performed in the:
   ❑ horizontal plane
   ❑ vertical plane
   ❑ diagonal plane

3) This exercise is to be performed:
   ❑ eyes open
   ❑ eyes closed

4) This exercise is to be performed:
   ❑ sitting, supported
   ❑ sitting, unsupported
   ❑ standing, supported and   ❑ feet shoulder-width apart   ❑ feet together
   ❑ standing, unsupported and   ❑ feet shoulder-width apart   ❑ feet together
   ❑ standing on a foam cushion

5) Hold the target card 12-18 inches in front of your eyes. Be sure you can focus on the letters on the card.

6) Keeping the cards *and* your head still, moving only your eyes, jump your eyes back and forth between the two cards. Take about one second per card and find a specific letter on which to focus on each card. Spell out words or sentences to vary the exercise.

7) Progress by moving the cards into the vertical plane and/or the diagonal plane as directed by your therapist. Try to keep increasing the speed at which your eyes are moving. Remember to keep the letters on each card in focus and use only your eyes, not your head, to move from one target card to the other.

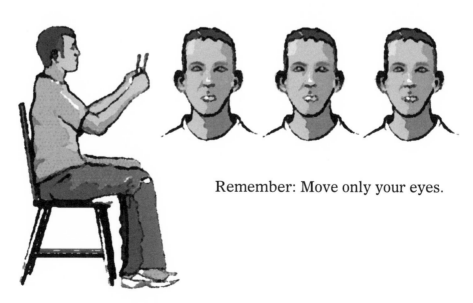

Remember: Move only your eyes.

OPTOKINETIC EYE MOVEMENTS

1) This exercise is to be performed _____ repeats.

2) This exercise is to be performed in the:
   □ horizontal plane
   □ vertical plane
   □ diagonal plane

3) This exercise is to be performed:
   □ eyes open
   □ eyes closed

4) This exercise is to be performed:
   □ sitting, supported
   □ sitting, unsupported
   □ standing, supported and □ feet shoulder-width apart □ feet together
   □ standing, unsupported and □ feet shoulder-width apart □ feet together
   □ standing on a foam cushion

5) Hold the optokinetic generator 12-18 inches in front of your eyes. Be sure you can focus on the letters on the card.

6) Keeping your head still, move the target slowly in front of your eyes, focusing on the center of the target.

7) Progress by moving the target into the vertical plane and/or the diagonal plane as directed by your therapist. Try to keep increasing the speed at which the target is moving. Remember to keep your head still. Have a partner look at your eye movements while doing the exercise. They should be "jumping" back and forth—a nystagmus movement.

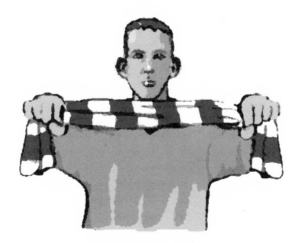

EXAMPLES OF EYE MOVEMENTS
FOR OCULAR MOTOR EXERCISES

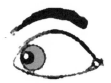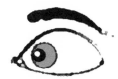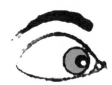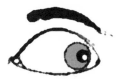

SIDE / SIDE

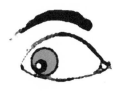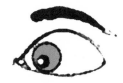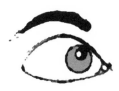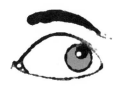

DIAGONALLY

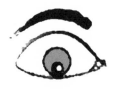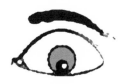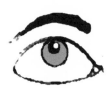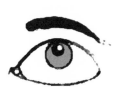

UP / DOWN

BRANDT-DAROFF EXERCISES— TO PREVENT THE RECURRENCE OF BPPV

If you develop neck or back pain, or if your position-provoked vertigo returns for more than a few seconds, stop doing the exercise and contact our office immediately.

1) Sit on the side of your bed with your feet flat on the floor.

2) Turn your head to the left, looking up toward the ceiling.

3) As rapidly as possible, fall to the right side, resting on your right shoulder. Turn your head slightly upward.

4) Stay in this position for as long as your symptoms last (or for 10-15 seconds if you do not have symptoms of vertigo or dizziness).

5) Sit up as rapidly as possible, pushing up with your left arm. Then turn your head to the right and fall down onto your left shoulder. Keep your head facing slightly upward.

6) Stay in this position for as long as your symptoms last (or for 10-15 seconds if you do not have symptoms of vertigo or dizziness).

7) Alternating sides, repeat the exercise a total of three times in both directions.

8) Do this exercise once daily.

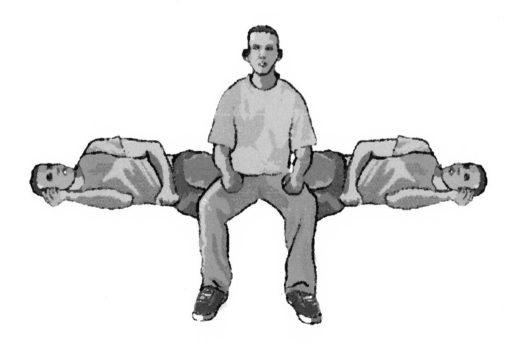

GAZE STABILIZATION WHILE STANDING ON A COMPLIANT SURFACE

1) This exercise is to be performed _____ repeats.

2) This exercise is to be performed in the:
   ❑ horizontal plane
   ❑ vertical plane
   ❑ diagonal plane

3) This exercise is to be performed:
   ❑ eyes open
   ❑ eyes closed

4) This exercise is to be performed:
   ❑ standing, unsupported and
   ❑ feet shoulder-width apart
   ❑ feet together

5) Hold the target card 12-18 inches in front of your eyes. Be sure you can focus on the letters on the card.

6) Keeping the card still and your eyes focused on the letters on the card, slowly move your head back and forth (horizontally), left and right. DO NOT MOVE YOUR HEAD SO FAST THAT THE LETTERS BECOME BLURRED OR OUT OF FOCUS!

7) Progress by moving your head in the vertical plane and/or the diagonal plane. Progress by placing the target card in the center of a busy visual background, such as a checkerboard. All progressions should be directed by your therapist. Try to keep increasing the speed that your head is moving. Remember to keep the letters on the card in focus—move only your head.

TOSSING AND CATCHING A BALL
(with or without a partner)

1) This exercise is to be performed____repeats.

2) This exercise is to be performed
   ❑ sitting, supported.
   ❑ sitting, unsupported.
   ❑ standing, supported and ❑ feet shoulder-width apart ❑ feet together
   ❑ standing, unsupported and ❑ feet shoulder-width apart ❑ feet together
   ❑ standing on a foam cushion.

3) Use a medium-sized ball for this exercise.
   (soccer ball, basketball, volleyball, etc.)

4) Keep your eyes fixed on the ball and move your head and eyes so that you are always looking at the ball.

5) Toss the ball into the air and catch it.

6) Bounce the ball off a wall at least 6 feet away and catch it.

7) Progress by moving from sitting to standing. Progress by moving to playing catch with someone else. Be sure to keep your eyes fixed on the ball at all times, using eye and head movements. All progressions should be directed by your therapist.

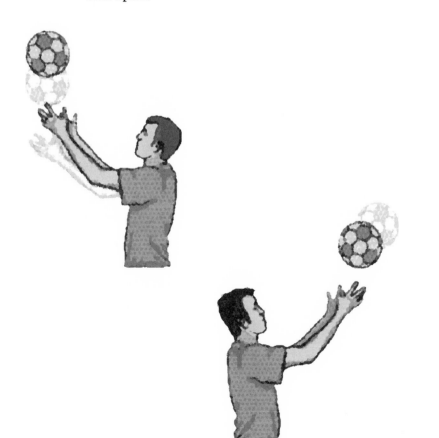
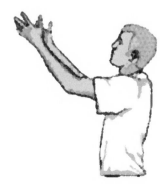

MOVING A BALL IN CIRCLES

1) This exercise is to be performed _____ repeats.

2) This exercise is to be performed:
   ❑ sitting, supported.
   ❑ sitting, unsupported.
   ❑ standing, supported and   ❑ feet shoulder-width apart   ❑ feet together.
   ❑ standing, unsupported and   ❑ feet shoulder-width apart   ❑ feet together.
   ❑ standing on a foam cushion.

3) Use a medium-sized ball for this exercise:
   soccer ball, basketball, volleyball, etc.

4) Keep your eyes fixed on the ball and move your head and eyes so that you are always looking at the ball.

5) Begin the exercise sitting. Move the ball in a large circle, over your head and down, almost sweeping the floor. Bend at the waist.

6) Progress by moving to a standing posture, feet shoulder-width apart. Again, make a big circle with the ball, moving your eyes and head so that you are always looking at the ball. Move the ball all the way over your head. Bend at the waist and the knees to move the ball downward, toward the floor. Progress by moving the ball faster and by narrowing your base of support by moving your feet closer together. All progressions should be directed by your therapist.

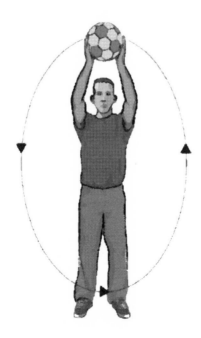

ANKLE SWAYS
(forward & back; left & right)

1) This exercise is to be performed _____ repeats.

2) This exercise is to be performed moving:
   ❑ forward & backward
   ❑ left & right

3) This exercise is to be performed:
   ❑ sitting, supported
   ❑ sitting, unsupported
   ❑ standing, supported and   ❑ feet shoulder-width apart   ❑ feet together
   ❑ standing, unsupported and   ❑ feet shoulder-width apart   ❑ feet together
   ❑ standing on a foam cushion

4) This exercise is done standing with your eyes focused on a target on the wall, MOVING ONLY AT YOUR ANKLES. (DO NOT bend at the shoulders, waist, hips, or knees.) Sway your body forward as far as you can, moving your weight onto the balls of your feet. Do not let your heels come up off the floor! Do not move so much that you lose your balance and need to take a step. Hold the position for 5 seconds, then move back to standing straight upright. Wait 5 seconds, then repeat.

5) Then do the exercise by swaying your body backward, moving your weight over your heels. MOVE ONLY AT YOUR ANKLES! Do not let your toes come up off the floor. Do not move so much that you lose your balance and need to take a step. Hold the position for 5 seconds, then move back to standing straight upright. Wait 5 seconds, then repeat.

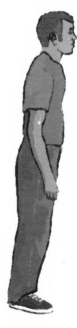

6) Sway to the left, moving your weight onto your left leg. Move as far as you can without your right leg coming off the floor. MOVE ONLY AT YOUR ANKLES! Do not move so much that you lose your balance and need to take a step. Hold the position for 5 seconds, then move back to standing straight upright. Wait 5 seconds, then repeat.

7) Sway to the right, moving your weight onto your right leg. Move as far as you can without your left leg coming off the floor. MOVE ONLY AT YOUR ANKLES! Do not move so much that you lose your balance and need to take a step. Hold the position for 5 seconds, then move back to standing straight upright. Wait 5 seconds, then repeat.

8) Progress by moving faster and by holding the leaning position for longer amounts of time. All progressions should be directed by your therapist.

ANKLE SWAYS
(circular)

1) This exercise is to be performed _____ repeats.

2) This exercise is to be performed:
   ❑ sitting, supported
   ❑ sitting, unsupported
   ❑ standing, supported and   ❑ feet shoulder-width apart   ❑ feet together
   ❑ standing, unsupported and   ❑ feet shoulder-width apart   ❑ feet together
   ❑ standing on a foam cushion

3) This exercise is done standing with your eyes focused on a target on the wall. MOVING ONLY AT YOUR ANKLES (DO NOT bend at the shoulders, waist, hips, or knees), sway your body in a large circle by shifting your weight over your feet. KEEP BOTH FEET FLAT ON THE FLOOR. Do not move so much that you lose your balance and need to take a step. Perform the exercise in both the clockwise and counterclockwise directions.

4) Progress by moving more quickly and by increasing the number of times the exercise is repeated.

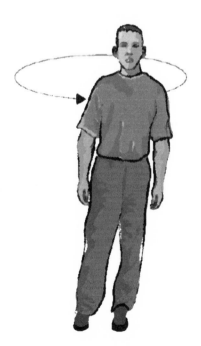

SIDE STEPPING

1) This exercise is to be performed _____ repeats.

2) This exercise is to be performed:
   ❑ standing, supported by a wall behind you
   ❑ standing, unsupported

3) Stand with your back against a flat wall for support. Standing still, with your feet together, slide your left leg to the side about 6-8 inches. Then slide your right leg to the left so that both feet are touching. Repeat.

4) Then, repeat the process by sliding your right leg to the side about 6-8 inches. Then, slide your left leg to the right so that both feet are touching. Repeat.

5) Progress by moving your feet farther apart each time, by moving more rapidly and by moving away from the wall. All progressions should be directed by your therapist.

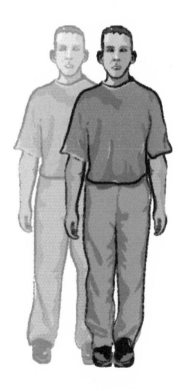

BODY ROLLING ALONG WALL

1) This exercise is to be performed _____ repeats.

2) This exercise is to be performed:
   ❑ standing, supported by a wall behind you.
   ❑ standing, unsupported.

3) This exercise is to be performed:
   ❑ eyes open.
   ❑ eyes closed.

4) Stand with your back against a flat wall for support. Slowly moving your feet, begin to turn your body and roll to the left, supported by the wall. Make one full 360 degree circle so that you end as you began, with your back to the wall.

5) Then, repeat the process but move in the opposite direction, rolling your body to the right, sliding your right leg to the side about 6-8 inches. Repeat the entire process.

6) Progress by moving your feet more rapidly and by moving away from the wall. Eventually, do the exercise with your back to the wall, but with your eyes closed. All progressions should be directed by your therapist.

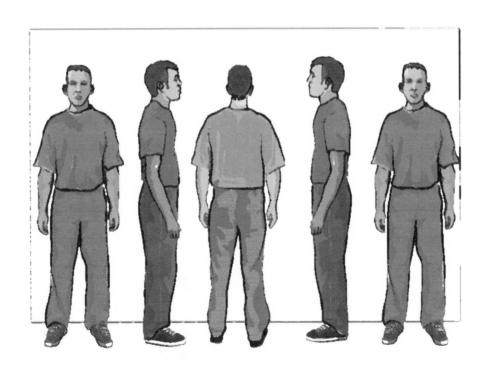

CROSS-OVER STEPPING

1) This exercise is to be performed ＿＿＿ repeats.

2) This exercise is to be performed:
   ❏ standing, supported by a wall behind you.
   ❏ standing, unsupported.

3) Stand with your back against a flat wall for support. Standing still, with your feet shoulder-width apart, move your right leg in front of your left, crossing over. Then, move your left leg behind the right, so that you are again standing with feet shoulder-width apart. Repeat.

4) Repeat the process by moving your left leg crossing in front of the right. Go back to the "feet shoulder-width apart stance" by moving the left leg behind the right. Repeat.

5) Progress by moving your feet farther apart each time, by moving more rapidly by starting from a stance with feet together and ankles touching, and by moving away from the wall. All progressions should be directed by your therapist.

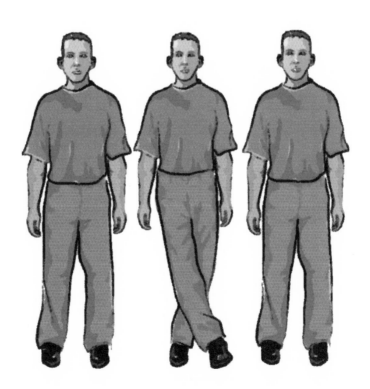

GAZE STABILIZATION WHILE WALKING

1) This exercise is to be performed _____ repeats.

2) With your eyes focused on a target directly in front of you, walk at least 10 feet toward the target. Try to walk as straight as you can, not veering left or right, but keeping your eyes fixed on the target. Repeat.

3) Progress by walking faster and by lowering the room lighting. Also, progress by placing the target in the center of a busy visual background, such as a checkerboard. All progressions should be directed by your therapist. Remember to keep the target in focus as you walk.

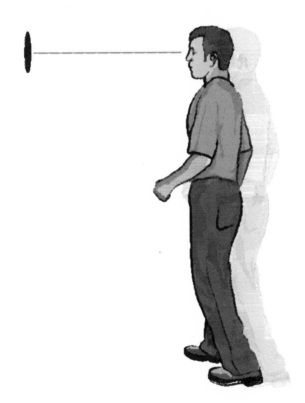

WALKING WITH HEAD MOVEMENTS

1) This exercise is to be performed _____ repeats.

2) This exercise is to be performed with head movements:
    ❑ in the horizontal plane.
    ❑ in the vertical plane.

3) Standing at the end of a hallway or an open area at least 10 feet long, begin walking. With every other step, move your head left and right: when your right foot is forward, move your head to the left; when your left foot is forward, move your head to the right. Try to walk as straight as you can, not veering left or right, but keeping your eyes fixed on the target. Repeat.

4) Progress by moving your head in the vertical direction, looking up or down every other step.

5) Progress by walking faster, by moving your head faster, and by lowering the room lighting. All progressions should be directed by your therapist.

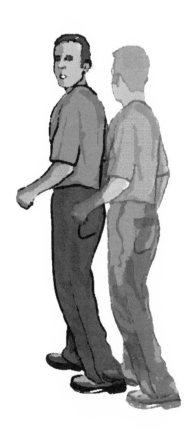

WALKING WITH QUICK STOPS

1) This exercise is to be performed _____ repeats.

2) This exercise is to be performed with:
   ❏ head movements in the horizontal plane
   ❏ head movements in the vertical plane
   ❏ no head movements—looking straight ahead

3) Standing at the end of a hallway or an open area at least 10 feet long, begin walking. Look at a target at the end of the hallway. After a few steps, stop abruptly. Use sway around your ankles to remain in balance and upright. Start walking again. Repeat.

4) Progress by having someone tell you when to stop when you are not expecting it. Progress by moving your head left and right. Progress by moving your head in the vertical direction, looking up or down every other step.

5) Progress by walking faster, by moving your head faster, and by lowering the room lighting. All progressions should be directed by your therapist.

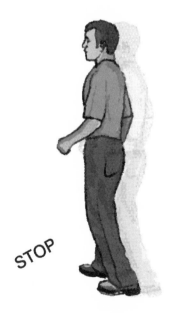

STOP

WALKING WITH QUICK STOPS & TURNS

1) This exercise is to be performed ____ repeats.

2) This exercise is to be performed with:
   ❑ head movements in the horizontal plane.
   ❑ head movements in the vertical plane.
   ❑ no head movements—looking straight ahead.

3) Standing at the end of a hallway or an open area at least 10 feet long, begin walking. Look at a target at the end of the hallway. After a few steps, stop abruptly. Use sway around your ankles to remain in balance and upright. Immediately turn around 180 degrees to the left, so you are now facing opposite the direction in which you began. Start walking again and repeat, this time turning to the right. Repeat each direction.

4) Progress by having someone tell you to stop when you are not expecting it. Your partner should then tell you "left" or "right" and you should turn in that direction. Progress by moving your head left and right. Progress by moving your head in the vertical direction, looking up or down every other step. Progress by turning a full 360 degree circle so you end up facing the same direction in which you started. Be careful to regain your full balance after you stop, before you begin to turn.

5) Progress by walking faster, by moving your head faster, and by lowering the room lighting. All progressions should be directed by your therapist.

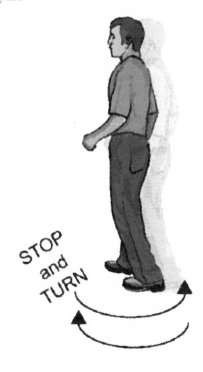

STOP and TURN

TANDEM WALKING

1) This exercise is to be performed _____ repeats.

2) This exercise is to be performed with:
   ❑ no head movements—looking straight ahead
   ❑ head movements in the horizontal plane
   ❑ head movements in the vertical plane

3) This exercise is to be performed with arms:
   ❑ stretched outward
   ❑ at your side
   ❑ folded across your chest

4) Standing at the end of a hallway or an open area at least 10 feet long, begin walking. Look at a target at the end of the hallway. Walk by placing one foot directly in front of the other, as though you were walking on a tightrope. Repeat.

5) Progress by moving your arms first to your sides and eventually folded across your chest in front of you.

6) Progress by moving your head left and right. Progress by moving your head in the vertical direction, looking up or down every other step.

7) Progress by walking faster, by moving your head faster, by stopping abruptly and restarting to walk, and by lowering the room lighting. All progressions should be directed by your therapist.

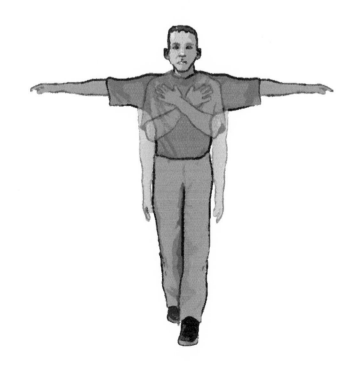

OBSTACLE COURSE

1) This entire battery of exercises is to be performed once daily.

2) Walk to the chair, sit in the chair, and stand up _____ times. Progress by sitting and bending over, and by walking around the chair several times each direction before sitting and standing.

3) Proceed to the box and step over it _____ times. Progress by bending over and picking up the box, lifting it overhead, and by picking up the box and turning 360 degrees before replacing it on the floor.

4) Go to the stool and walk a circle around it _____ times each direction. Progress by sitting down on the stool and stand up after you walk around it each time, pick up the stool and move it several feet before sitting down and standing, and then tandem walk around the stool.

5) Lastly, pick up the ball and move it in a large circle, from overhead to sweeping the floor by bending at the waist and knees. Use head-and-eye movements to keep your gaze fixated on the ball at all times. Progress by tossing the ball in the air and catching it, bounce it off the floor or a wall, and play "catch" with a partner.

Remember, all progressions should be directed by your therapist.

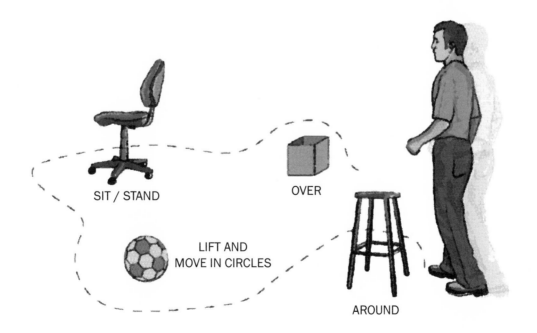

SIT / STAND

OVER

LIFT AND
MOVE IN CIRCLES

AROUND